Pediatric Pulseless Arrest

Verify pulselessnesss, start CPR. *Consider* underlying causes listed below.

VF or pulseless VT

Defibrillate up to 3 times: 2J/kg, then 2-4 J/kg, then 4J/kg
Continue CPR. Secure airway, ventilate with 100% O_2.
Obtain IV or IO access.

↓

Epinephrine Q 3-5min
IV: 0.01 mg/kg (1:10,000, 0.1 ml/kg)
ET: 0.1 mg/kg (1:1000, 0.1 ml/kg).

↓

Defibrillate 4J/kg 30-60sec later

↓

Aminodarone 5 mg/kg IV; or lidocaine 1 mg/kg IV. If torsades or hypomag present, magnesium 25-50 mg/kg IV.

↓

Defibrillate 4J/kg 30-60sec later

↓

Epinephrine 1:1000 0.1 mg/kg IV/ET. *Consider* dosing up to 0.2 mg/kg of 1:1000.

↓

Defibrillate 4J/kg 30-60sec later

↓

Verify ET placement, paddle position/contact. *Consider* alternative meds/buffers.

Asystole/PEA

Continue CPR.
Secure airway.
Ventilate with 100% O_2.
Obtain IV or IO access.

↓

Epinephrine
IV: 0.01 mg/kg
(1:10,000, 0.1 ml/kg);
ET: 0.1 mg/kg
(1:1000, 0.1 ml/kg)

↓

Epinephrine
1:1000 0.1 mg/kg IV/ET.
Consider dosing up to
0.2 mg/kg of 1:1000.
Repeat Q 3-5min.

↓

Verify ET placement.
Consider alternative
meds & buffers.

↓

Diagnose, treat causes below.

Causes: severe hypoxia, hypovolemia, hypothermia, acidosis, tension pneumo, cardiac tamponade, electrolyte imbalance, OD, PE.

For Pediatric Bradycardia protocol, see page ii
For Neonatal Resuscitation protocol, see inside back cover
For Pediatric Fever protocols, see p. 323
For adult ACLS protocols, see p. 324

Pediatric Bradycardia

Usually caused by hypoxia. *Other causes:* hypovolemia, tension pneumo, electrolyte imbalance, heart transplant, acidosis, head injury, OD, hypothermia, cardiac tamponade, increased vagal tone*, heart block*.

Assess ABC's & VS, give 100% O$_2$, obtain IV or IO access and ECG

Severe cardiorespiratory compromise?

No

Yes

Observe, support ABC's, consider transfer to ALS facility

Oxygenate, ventilate, intubate. Do chest compressions if HR <60 BPM in an infant/child with poor perfusion.

Epinephrine Q 3-5min
IV: 0.01 mg/kg (1:10,000, 0.1 ml/kg)
ET: 0.1 mg/kg (1:1000, 0.1 ml/kg)

*Atropine 0.02 mg/kg IV/ET, dose range is minimum 0.1 mg to max 0.5 mg for child, max 1.0 mg for adolescent

Consider pacing

Consider epinephrine or dopamine infusions

If arrest occurs: go to *Pediatric Pulseless Arrest* protocol

*Give atropine first for suspected increase in vagal tone or AV block

For Pediatric Pulseless arrest protocol, see page i
For Neonatal Resuscitation protocol, see inside back cover
For Pediatric Fever protocols, see p. 323
For adult ACLS protocols, see p. 324

Detroit Receiving Hospital

EMERGENCY MEDICINE HANDBOOK

Fifth Edition

Editor: William A. Berk, MD

F.A. Davis Company • Philadelphia

F. A. Davis Company
1915 Arch Street
Philadelphia, PA 19103
www.fadavis.com

Printed in Canada

Last digit indicates print number: 10 9 8 7 6 5 4 3 2 1

Acquisitions Editor: Andrew McPhee
Manager, Content Development: Deborah Thorp
Manager of Art & Design: Carolyn O'Brien

As new scientific information becomes available through basic and clinical research, recommended treatments and drug therapies undergo changes. The author(s) and publisher have done everything possible to make this book accurate, up to date, and in accord with accepted standards at the time of publication. The author(s), editors, and publisher are not responsible for errors or omissions or for consequences from application of the book, and make no warranty, expressed or implied, in regard to the contents of the book. Any practice described in this book should be applied by the reader in accordance with professional standards of care used in regard to the unique circumstances that may apply in each situation. The reader is advised always to check product information (package inserts) for changes and new information regarding dose and contraindications before administering any drug. Caution is especially urged when using new or infrequently ordered drugs.

Editor-in-Chief
William A. Berk, MD
Vice-Chief, Emergency Department
Detroit Receiving Hospital
Associate Professor of Emergency Medicine
Wayne State University
Detroit, Michigan

Associate Editor
Phillip D. Levy, MD
Assistant Professor of Emergency Medicine
Wayne State University
Emergency Department
Detroit Receiving Hospital
Detroit, Michigan

Senior Editor for Drug Therapy and Pharmacy
Elizabeth Clements, PharmD
Clinical Pharmacy Specialist, Emergency Medicine
Spectrum Health
Detroit, Michigan

The *Detroit Receiving Hospital Emergency Medicine Handbook* was conceived as a means of compiling, in a format that was easy to use and carry, the information most frequently used, but not memorized, by emergency medicine practitioners.

The *Handbook* has evolved from its first edition, through its daily use in the challenging environment of the Detroit Receiving Hospital Emergency Department, a nationally renowned trauma and emergency center. Changes through successive editions have been the result of our own experiences using the book in actual practice, as well as the experiences of our residents, nurses, and physicians' assistants. In addition, the physicians and pharmacists who serve as *Handbook* editors also work in pediatric emergency centers and suburban and rural EDs. Their experiences have been incorporated throughout the *Handbook*.

In this latest edition, we have strived to focus on information that reflects the rapid evolution of emergency medicine as a specialty. The *Handbook* features up-to-date information on adult and pediatric medication dosing, trauma care, toxicology, pediatric emergency care, internal medicine including cardiology, and the treatment of specific diseases. As well, we cover the latest advances in ACLS, ATLS, RSI, and PALS, among other emergency medicine protocols.

We've reorganized information in this edition to help you find what you're looking for more quickly and more easily than ever before. As always, this *Handbook* emphasizes the clinical application of knowledge through the use of standard treatment protocols, drug dosing, diagnostic aids, and nationally accepted guidelines, presented in a space-saving format. We've worked hard to present this information in the clearest and most time-efficient way possible. That's why you'll find compact and consistently structured tables, well laid-out algorithms, helpful charts, and other key pieces of information throughout the book.

Aside from being proud of the information we've included, I'm also proud of the hard decisions our editors have made about what information *not* to include. By focusing on the *necessary,* we've created what I think is, ounce-for-ounce, the most powerful management aid emergency medicine practitioners can carry with them as they make their daily rounds in the ED.

We always welcome input from our users. If you have an idea for the sixth edition, please contact us. If you're the first to think of it and we incorporate it into our next edition, we'll send you a free copy. In the meantime, please enjoy this completely updated edition. And don't forget to pass on our Order Card in the back to a colleague!

Section Editors

Toxicology . . . . .Suzanne R. White, MD
Associate Professor of Emergency Medicine
Wayne State University
Emergency Department
Detroit Receiving Hospital
Detroit, Michigan

Pediatrics . . . . .Matthew Denenberg, MD
Pediatric Emergency Physician
Assistant Clinical Professor, Michigan State University
Spectrum Health–Devos Children's Hospital
Grand Rapids, Michigan

Drug Dosing Table Editors . . . . Christine Ahrens, PharmD
Clinical Pharmacy Specialist – Neuro-ICU
Cleveland Clinic Foundation
Department of Pharmacy Services
Cleveland, Ohio

Wanda Blount, RPh
Clinical Pharmacist
Detroit Receiving Hospital
Department of Pharmacy Services
Detroit, Michigan

George Delgado, Jr., PharmD
Coordinator, Emergency Pharmacy Services
Clinical Pharmacy Specialist – Emergency Medicine
Detroit Receiving Hospital
Department of Pharmacy Services
Detroit, Michigan

Pamela Lada, PharmD
Clinical Pharmacy Specialist – Emergency Medicine
Boston Medical Center
Department of Pharmacy Services
Boston, Massachusetts

Jamie Shaskos, PharmD
Clinical Pharmacist
Detroit Receiving Hospital
Department of Pharmacy Services
Detroit, Michigan

Dana Staat, PharmD
Assistant Professor, Pharmacy Practice
Ferris State University College of Pharmacy
St. Mary's Health Care
Grand Rapids, Michigan

Stephen Zbikowski, RPh
Clinical Pharmacist
Detroit Receiving Hospital
Department of Pharmacy Services
Detroit, Michigan

CONTENTS

ACLS PROTOCOLS

1. Comprehensive Algorithm for Pulselessness

Person collapses
Possible cardiac arrest
Assess responsiveness

Unresponsive

Begin Primary ABCD Survey
(Begin BLS Algorithm)
Activate emergency response
Call for defibrillator
A Assess breathing (open airway, *look, listen, and feel*)

Not breathing
B Give 2 slow breaths
C Assess pulse; if no pulse, then
C Start chest compressions
D Attach monitor/defibrillator when available

No pulse
CPR continues
Assess rhythm

(continued on following page)

ACLS PROTOCOLS *(cont.)*

Comprehensive Algorithm for Pulselessness
(continued)

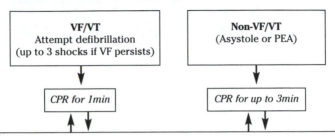

| **VF/VT**
Attempt defibrillation
(up to 3 shocks if VF persists) | **Non-VF/VT**
(Asystole or PEA) |

CPR for 1min   *CPR for up to 3min*

Secondary ABCD Survey
- **Airway:** attempt to place airway device
- **Breathing:** confirm and secure airway device, ventilations, oxygenation
- **Circulation:** gain intravenous access; give adrenergic agent; consider antiarrhythmics, buffer agents, pacing
  Non-VF/VT patients:
  —**Epinephrine:** 1mg IV, repeat every 3-5min
  VF/VT patients:
  —**Vasopressin:** 40U IV single dose, 1 time only; *or*
  —**Epinephrine:** 1mg IV, repeat dose every 3-5min (if no response 10min after single dose of **vasopressin,** may start **epinephrine,** 1mg IV push; repeat every 3-5min)
- **Differential Diagnosis:** search for and treat reversible causes

2. Ventricular Fibrillation/Pulseless VT Algorithm

Focus: basic CPR and defibrillation
Check responsiveness
Activate emergency response system
Call for defibrillator

(continued on following page)

A **Airway:** open the airway
B **Breathing:** provide positive-pressure ventilations
C **Circulation:** give chest compressions
D **Defibrillation:** assess for and shock VF/pulseless VT, up to 3 times (200J, 200-300J, 360J, or equivalent *biphasic*) if necessary

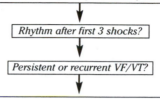

Rhythm after first 3 shocks?

Persistent or recurrent VF/VT?

Secondary ABCD Survey
Focus: more advanced assessments and treatments
A **Airway:** place airway device as soon as possible
B **Breathing:** confirm airway device placement by exam plus confirmation device; purpose-made tube holders preferred
B **Breathing:** confirm effective oxygenation and ventilations
C **Circulation:** establish IV access
C **Circulation:** identify rhythm and monitor
C **Circulation:** administer drugs appropriate for rhythm and condition
D **Differential Diagnosis:** search for and treat identified reversible causes

Epinephrine: 1mg IV push every 3-5min; *or*
Vasopressin: 40U IV, **single dose,** 1 time only

(continued on following page)

ACLS PROTOCOLS *(cont.)*

Ventricular Fibrillation/Pulseless VT Algorithm
(continued)

Resume attempts to defibrillate
1 × 360 (or equivalent *biphasic*) within 30-60sec

Consider antiarrhythmics:
Amiodarone (IIb)
Lidocaine (indeterminate)
Magnesium (IIb if hypomagnesemic state)
Procainamide (IIb for intermittent/recurrent VF/VT)
Consider buffers

Resume attempts to defibrillate

3. Pulseless Electrical Activity Algorithm (PEA)

PEA = rhythm on monitor without detectable pulse

Primary ABCD Survey
Focus: *basic CPR and defibrillation*
Check responsiveness
Activate emergency response system
Call for defibrillator
A Airway: open the airway
B Breathing: provide positive-pressure ventilations
C Circulation: give chest compressions
D Defibrillation: assess for and shock VF/pulseless VT

(continued on following page)

Secondary ABCD Survey
Focus: *more advanced assessments and treatments*

A **Airway:** place airway device as soon as possible

B **Breathing:** confirm airway device placement by exam plus confirmation device

B **Breathing:** secure airway device; purpose-made tube holders preferred

B **Breathing:** confirm effective oxygenation and ventilations

C **Circulation:** establish IV access

C **Circulation:** identify rhythm, and monitor

C **Circulation:** administer drugs appropriate for rhythm and condition

C **Circulation:** assess for occult blood flow ("pseudo-EMD")

D **Differential Diagnosis:** search for and treat reversible causes

Review for most frequent causes

- Hypovolemia
- Hypoxia
- Hydrogen ion (acidosis)
- Hyper-/hypokalemia
- Hypothermia
- "Tablets" (drug OD, accidents)
- Tamponade, cardiac
- Tension pneumothorax
- Thrombosis, coronary (ACS)
- Thrombosis, pulmonary (PE)

Epinephrine: 1mg IV push, repeat every 3-5min

Atropine: 1mg IV (if PEA rate is **slow**),
repeat every 3-5min as needed, to a total dose of 0.04mg/kg

ACLS PROTOCOLS *(cont.)*

4. Asystole

Primary ABCD Survey
Focus: basic CPR and defibrillation

Check responsiveness
Activate emergency response system
Call for defibrillator
A Airway: open the airway
B Breathing: provide positive-pressure ventilations
C Circulation: give chest compressions; confirm asystole
D Defibrillation: assess for and shock VF/pulseless VT

Secondary ABCD Survey
Focus: more advanced assessments and treatments

A Airway: place airway device as soon as possible
B Breathing: confirm airway device placement by exam plus confirmation device
B Breathing: secure airway device; purpose-made tube holders preferred
B Breathing: confirm effective oxygenation and ventilations
C Circulation: confirm true asystole
C Circulation: establish IV access
C Circulation: identify rhythm and monitor
C Circulation: administer drugs appropriate for rhythm and condition
D Differential Diagnosis: search for and treat reversible causes

---

Transcutaneous pacing
If considered, pace immediately

(continued on following page)

Epinephrine: 1mg IV push, repeat every 3-5min

Atropine: 1mg IV, repeat every 3-5min as needed, to a total dose of 0.04mg/kg

Asystole persists
Withhold or cease resuscitation efforts? Consider:
- What is the quality of resuscitation?
- Atypical clinical features present?
- Support for ceasing efforts—protocols in place?

5. Bradycardia

- ***Slow*** (absolute bradycardia = rate <60bpm)
  or
- ***Relatively slow*** (rate less than expected in relation to underlying condition or cause)

Primary ABCD Survey
- Assess ABCs
- Secure airway non-invasively
- Ensure monitor/defibrillator is available

(continued on following page)

ACLS PROTOCOLS *(cont.)*

Bradycardia

(continued)

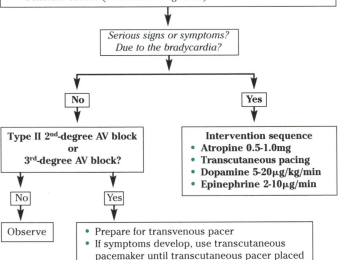

Secondary ABCD Survey
- Assess secondary ABCs (invasive airway management needed?)
- Oxygen, IV access, monitor, fluids
- Vital signs, pulse oximeter, monitor BP
- Obtain and review 12-lead ECG
- Obtain and review portable chest x-ray
- Problem-focused history
- Problem-focused physical examination
- Consider causes (differential diagnoses)

Serious signs or symptoms?
Due to the bradycardia?

No

Yes

Type II 2nd-degree AV block
or
3rd-degree AV block?

Intervention sequence
- **Atropine 0.5-1.0mg**
- **Transcutaneous pacing**
- **Dopamine 5-20µg/kg/min**
- **Epinephrine 2-10µg/min**

No

Yes

Observe

- Prepare for transvenous pacer
- If symptoms develop, use transcutaneous pacemaker until transcutaneous pacer placed

6. Tachycardia*

With serious signs and symptoms related to the tachycardia

If ventricular rate is >150bpm, prepare for **immediate cardioversion.** May give brief trial of medications on basis of specific arrhythmias. Immediate cardioversion is generally not needed if heart rate is ≤150bpm.

Have available at bedside:
- Oxygen saturation monitor
- Suction device
- IV line
- Intubation equipment

Premedicate whenever possible

Synchronized cardioversion
- Ventricular tachycardia
- Paroxysmal supraventricular tachycardia
- Atrial fibrillation
- Atrial flutter

Stepwise increases as follows: 100J, 200J, 300J, 360J monophasic energy dose (or clinically equivalent biphasic energy dose). **If delays in synchronization occur and clinical condition is critical, go immediately to unsynchronized shocks.**

See also algorithms for Stable Ventricular Tachycardia, p. 14, and Narrow Complex Supraventricular Tachycardia, p. 10.

ACLS PROTOCOLS *(cont.)*

7. Narrow-Complex Supraventricular Tachycardia, Stable

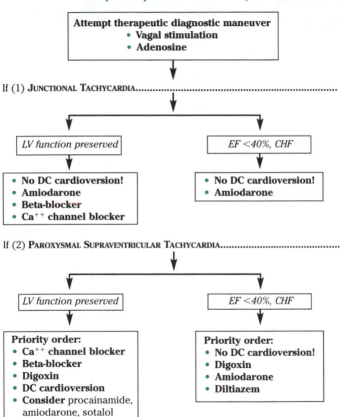

Attempt therapeutic diagnostic maneuver
- **Vagal stimulation**
- **Adenosine**

If (1) JUNCTIONAL TACHYCARDIA...

LV function preserved

- **No DC cardioversion!**
- **Amiodarone**
- **Beta-blocker**
- **Ca⁺⁺ channel blocker**

EF <40%, CHF

- **No DC cardioversion!**
- **Amiodarone**

If (2) PAROXYSMAL SUPRAVENTRICULAR TACHYCARDIA..

LV function preserved

Priority order:
- **Ca⁺⁺ channel blocker**
- **Beta-blocker**
- **Digoxin**
- **DC cardioversion**
- **Consider** procainamide, amiodarone, sotalol

EF <40%, CHF

Priority order:
- **No DC cardioversion!**
- **Digoxin**
- **Amiodarone**
- **Diltiazem**

(continued on following page)

If (3) ECTOPIC OR MULTIFOCAL ATRIAL TACHYCARDIA..

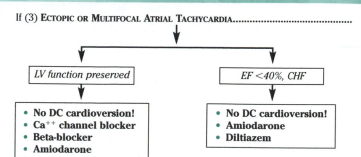

LV function preserved

- **No DC cardioversion!**
- **Ca^{++} channel blocker**
- **Beta-blocker**
- **Amiodarone**

EF <40%, CHF

- **No DC cardioversion!**
- **Amiodarone**
- **Diltiazem**

8. Tachycardia Overview Algorithm

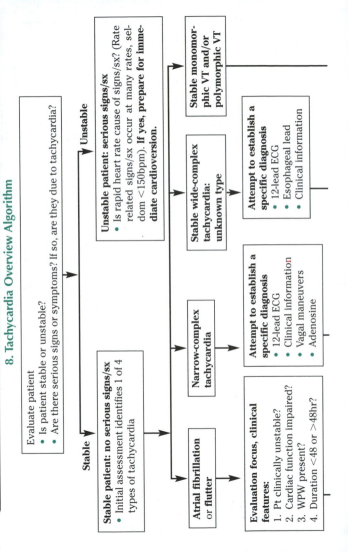

Evaluate patient
- Is patient stable or unstable?
- Are there serious signs or symptoms? If so, are they due to tachycardia?

Stable

Unstable

Stable patient: no serious signs/sx
- Initial assessment identifies 1 of 4 types of tachycardia

Unstable patient: serious signs/sx
- Is rapid heart rate cause of signs/sx? (Rate related signs/sx occur at many rates, seldom <150bpm). **If yes, prepare for immediate cardioversion.**

Atrial fibrillation or flutter

Narrow-complex tachycardia

Stable wide-complex tachycardia: unknown type

Stable monomorphic VT and/or polymorphic VT

Evaluation focus, clinical features:
1. Pt clinically unstable?
2. Cardiac function impaired?
3. WPW present?
4. Duration <48 or >48hr?

Attempt to establish a specific diagnosis
- 12-lead ECG
- Clinical information
- Vagal maneuvers
- Adenosine

Attempt to establish a specific diagnosis
- 12-lead ECG
- Esophageal lead
- Clinical information

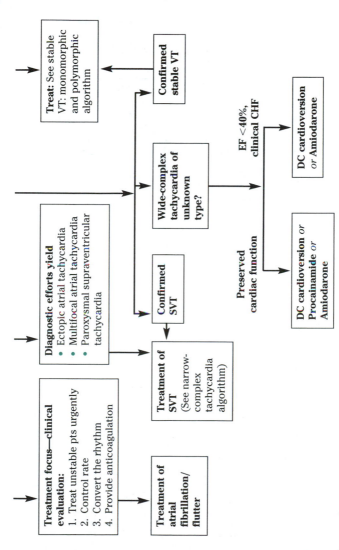

Treatment focus—clinical evaluation:
1. Treat unstable pts urgently
2. Control rate
3. Convert the rhythm
4. Provide anticoagulation

Treatment of atrial fibrillation/flutter

Diagnostic efforts yield
- Ectopic atrial tachycardia
- Multifocal atrial tachycardia
- Paroxysmal supraventricular tachycardia

Confirmed SVT

Treatment of SVT (See narrow-complex tachycardia algorithm)

Wide-complex tachycardia of unknown type?

Confirmed stable VT

Treat: See stable VT: monomorphic and polymorphic algorithm

Preserved cardiac function

EF <40%, clinical CHF

DC cardioversion or **Procainamide** or **Amiodarone**

DC cardioversion or **Amiodarone**

13

9. Stable Ventricular Tachycardia

Monomorphic or polymorphic?
Note: **may go directly to cardioversion**

Monomorphic VT
• Is cardiac function impaired?

NL LV function

Medications: any 1 med
• Procainamide
• Sotalol
Others acceptable
• Amiodarone
• Lidocaine

Poor EF

Normal baseline QT interval
• Treat ischemia
• Correct electrolytes
Medications: any 1 med
• Beta-blockers
• Lidocaine
• Amiodarone
• Procainamide
• Sotalol

Polymorphic VT
• Is QT baseline interval prolonged?

NL baseline QT

Prolonged baseline QT interval
(suggests torsades)

Long baseline QT interval
• Treat ischemia
• Correct abnormal electrolytes
Medications: any 1 med
• Magnesium
• Overdrive pacing
• Isoproterenol
• Phenytoin
• Lidocaine

(*Either* amiodarone 150mg IV bolus over 10min *or* lidocaine 0.5–0.75mg/kg IV push); then **synchronized cardioversion**

RAPID-SEQUENCE INTUBATION (RSI)

General Considerations

1. **Pre-oxygenate:** if possible, allow the patient to spontaneously breathe 100% O_2 for 3-5min. Do not bag a patient who is breathing adequately, as this may induce aspiration.
2. **Pre-treatment:** it may be desirable to omit all or part of this step under certain circumstances. For example, hypotensive patients do not require *lidocaine,* and waiting for a defasciculating dose to take effect may be impractical in critically ill or injured patients.
   * *Vecuronium* 0.01mg/kg *or rocuronium* 0.06-0.1mg/kg IVP (*defasciculating dose*); *and/or*
   * *Lidocaine* 1.5mg/kg rapidly IV (*may blunt rise in intracranial [IC] pressure in head-injured patients*); *and/or*
   * *Fentanyl* 3.0µg/kg IVP (*also useful in head-injured patients*); *and/or*
   * *Atropine* 0.02mg/kg IVP recommended for children, 1.0mg IVP optional for adults (*reduces bradycardia and secretions*).
3. **Sedation:** an essential step, as it ensures the patient will not be awake while paralyzed. With the exception of *sodium thiopental* (which is very rapid acting and therefore a good choice when time is essential), sedatives should be administered at least 60sec before paralyzing agents. Choice of medication is based on the specific clinical situation.

Primary Choices

   * *Etomidate* 0.2–0.4mg/kg IVP (may cause myoclonus, pain on injection, adrenal suppression; it has little effect on ventilation or hemodynamics, and lowers IC pressure — good for hypotensive or head-injured patients; giving 2-3mg 1min before larger dose reduces myoclonus), *or*
   * *Sodium thiopental* 2–5mg/kg IVP (helpful in head-injured or hypertensive patients; avoid if hypotension/asthma present).

Secondary Choices

   * *Fentanyl* 1.5-5.0µg/kg IVP (causes respiratory depression, rigidity, bradycardia, laryngospasm, and nausea and vomiting; blunts pressor response to intubation; maximum dose in trauma patients: 3µg/kg); *or*

(continued on following page)

RAPID-SEQUENCE INTUBATION (RSI) *(cont.)*

- *Ketamine* 1.0-1.5mg/kg IVP (may be useful in status asthmaticus; avoid in head injuries and hypovolemic trauma cases); *or*
- *Propofol* 1.0-2.5mg/kg IVP (may cause hypotension or respiratory depression; rapid recovery time, lowers ICP).

4. *Paralytic Agent*

Primary Choice

- *Succinylcholine* 1.0-1.5mg/kg (*young children, up to 2mg/kg*) IVP (short duration of action means it is most often the agent of choice; it is safe and effective in cases of head injuries but should be avoided if hyperkalemia is possible; if a ruptured globe is present, use a defasiculating dose of *vecuronium* or *rocuronium* [see under #2]).

Secondary Choice

- *Rocuronium* 0.6-1.2mg/kg IVP (onset/duration of action are slightly longer than *succinylcholine;* unlike other non-depolarizing agents, it has few effects on hemodynamics and virtually no associated bronchospasm; it is therefore the non-depolarizing agent of choice for RSI).

DETROIT RECEIVING HOSPITAL RAPID-SEQUENCE INTUBATION PROTOCOL

Time 0-3.0 minutes	*Pre-oxygenate (continue until patient intubated):* Assemble drugs and prepare for intubation
Time 3.0-3.5 minutes	*Pre-treat if desired or needed with lidocaine, precurarizing agents, fentanyl, atropine*
Time 3.5-4.0 minutes	*Administer sedation, allow 1-2min for effect*
Time 5.0-5.5 minutes	*Administer paralytic agent and wait 1min:* Perform Sellick's maneuver (gentle cricoid pressure) Administer paralytic agent
Time 6.5 minutes	*Intubate*

NORMAL RESTING HEMODYNAMIC VALUES

Pressure/resistance	Range
Central venous	0-6cm H_2O
Right atrial	0-5mm Hg
Pulmonary vascular resistance	255-285dyne-sec/cm^5-m^2
Right ventricular	
Systolic	15-30mm Hg
Diastolic	0-8mm Hg
Pulmonary arterial	
Systolic	15-30mm Hg
Diastolic	3-12mm Hg
Pulmonary wedge	3-15mm Hg
Left atrial	2-12mm Hg
Left ventricular	
Systolic	100-140mm Hg
Diastolic	3-12mm Hg
Systemic vascular resistance	1970-2390dyne-sec/cm^5-m^2

TIMI RISK SCORE FOR UNSTABLE ANGINA/NON–ST ELEVATION MI

Variables	Points
Age ≥65	1
≥3 CAD RF: HTN, cholesterol, DM, active smoker, +FH	1
Known CAD (stenosis ≥50%)	1
ASA use in past 7d	1
Severe angina (≥2 events in past 24h)	1
Elevated serum cardiac biomarkers	1
ST deviation ≥0.5mm	1

Outcome at 14 Days (%)

Risk Score	Death or MI	Death, MI, or Urgent Revascularization
0/1	3	5
2	3	8
3	5	13
4	7	20
5	12	26
6/7	19	41

Adapted from: *JAMA* 2000; 284:835.

PRETEST PROBABILITY OF DVT

Clinical Feature	Points
Active cancer (treatment ongoing, within 6 months, or palliative)	1
Paralysis, paresis, or recent immobilization of lower extremity	1
Recently bedridden for >3d or major surgery within 4wk	1
Tenderness along distribution of deep venous system	1
Entire leg swollen	1
Calf swelling with circumference disparity >3cm (measured 10cm distal to tibial tuberosity)	1
Pitting edema, greater in symptomatic leg	1
Collateral superficial veins visible (non-varicose)	1
Alternative diagnosis as likely as or greater than that of DVT	−2

Interpretation of Score

Score	Probability of DVT	DVT Prevalence (%)
≤0	Low	3
1 or 2	Moderate	17
≥3	High	75

Adapted from: *Lancet* 1997; 350:1795.

PRETEST PROBABILITY OF PULMONARY EMBOLISM

Clinical Feature	Points
Suspected DVT	3
An alternative diagnosis is less likely than PE	3
Heart rate >100 beats per minute	1.5
Immobilization or surgery in the previous 4 weeks	1.5
Previous DVT or PE	1.5
Hemoptysis	1
Malignancy (on treatment, treated in the past 6 months, or palliative)	1

Interpretation of Score

Score	Probability of PE	PE Prevalence (%)
0-2 points	Low	3.6
3-6 points	Moderate	20.5
>6 points	High	66.7

Adapted from: *Thromb Haemost* 2000; 83:416.

COMMUNITY-ACQUIRED PNEUMONIA PREDICTION RULE (PORT SCORE)

Step 1

Start with these questions:

1. Is the patient >50yr old?
2. Does the patient have neoplastic disease *or* congestive heart failure *or* cerebrovascular disease *or* renal disease *or* liver disease?
3. Does the patient have altered mental status *or* pulse ≥125bpm *or* respiratory rate ≥30/min *or* systolic blood pressure ≤90mm Hg *or* temperature <35°C or ≥40°C?

If answer to all is no, assign the patient to Risk Class I.
If answer to any is yes, proceed to step 2.

Step 2

Variable	Points Assigned
Demographic factor	
Age	
Men	Age (yr)
Women	Age (yr)–10
Nursing home resident	+10
Coexistent illnesses	
Neoplastic disease	+30
Liver disease	+20
Congestive heart failure	+10
Cerebrovascular disease	+10
Renal disease	+10

Variable	Points Assigned
Physical examination findings	
Altered mental status	+20
Respiratory rate ≥30/min	+20
Systolic blood pressure ≤90mm Hg	+20
Temperature <35°C or ≥40°C	+15
Pulse ≥125bpm	+10
Laboratory and radiographic findings	
Arterial pH <7.35	+30
Blood urea nitrogen ≥30mg/dl (11 mmol/liter)	+20
Sodium <130mmol/liter	+20

(continued on following page)

COMMUNITY-ACQUIRED PNEUMONIA PREDICTION RULE (PORT SCORE) *(cont.)*

Glucose ≥250mg/dl (14 mmol/liter)	+10
Hematocrit <30%	+10
Partial pressure of arterial O_2 <60mm Hg or O_2 saturation <90%	+10
Pleural effusion	+10

Interpretation of Score

Point Total (Score)	Risk Class	Mortality (%)	Care Locale
None calculated	I	0.1-0.4	Outpatient
≤70	II	0.6-0.7	Outpatient
71-90	III	0.9-2.8	Inpatient
91-130	IV	8.2-9.3	Inpatient
>130	V	27.0-31.1	Inpatient

Adapted from: *N Engl J Med* 1997; 336:243.

DENTAL ANATOMY

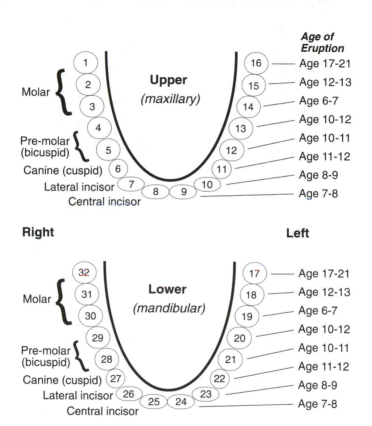

Figure 2–1   Dental anatomy.

SENSORY DERMATOMES

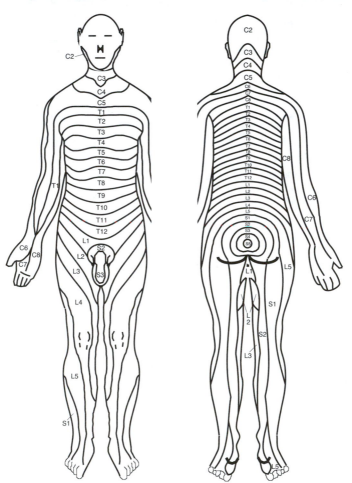

Figure 2–2 Sensory dermatomes.

SPINAL CORD LEVELS: SENSORY AND MOTOR

Sensory		Motor	
C2	Occiput	C1-C4	Flexion, extension, rotation of neck
C3	Thyroid cartilage		
C4	Suprasternal notch	C3-C5	Spontaneous breathing
C5	Below clavicle	C3-C5	Shrugging of shoulders
C6	Thumb	C5-C6	Elbow flexion
C7	Index finger	C6-C8	Elbow extension
C8	Small finger	C6-C8	Hand extension
T4	Nipple line	C6-C8	Finger extension
T10	Umbilicus	C7-T1	Hand flexion
L1	Inguinal ligament	C7-T1	Finger flexion
L2-L3	Medial thigh	L1-L3	Hip flexion
L4	Knee	L2-L4	Leg extension
L5	Lateral calf	L3-L4	Hip adduction
S1	Lateral foot	L4-S2	Hip abduction
S2-S4	Perineum	L4-S1	Foot dorsiflexion
S2	Gluteus maximus	L5-S2	Foot plantar flexion
S3-4	Anal sphincter	L5-S1	Toe extension
		L5-S2	Toe flexion
		S2-S4	Sphincter tone

Reflexes

CN VII	Corneal	L2-L4	Patellar
CN IX	Gag	S1	Achilles
C5-C6	Biceps	S1-S2	Plantar
C6-C7	Triceps	S2-S4	Bulbocavernosus
T1-T2	Ciliospinal	S4-S5	Anal
L1	Cremasteric		

HAND MOTOR EXAM

Nerve = nerve innervation; **M** = median; **U** = ulnar; **R** = radial

Extrinsic Hand Flexors

Muscle(s)	Nerve	Test
Flexor pollicis longus	M	Flexion of the distal phalanx of the thumb.
Flexor digitorum profundus	M, U*	Test 2nd to 5th separately. MCP and PIP of tested finger held in extension by examiner while patient flexes DIP joint.
Flexor digitorum superficialis	M	Test 2nd to 5th separately. Untested fingers are held in extension by examiner while patient flexes PIP joint.
Flexor carpi radialis	M	While the patient, making a fist, flexes the wrist against resistance, these tendons are palpated respectively in the radial, central, and ulnar regions of the volar wrist.
Palmaris longus	M	
Flexor carpi ulnaris	U	

*Thumb and index fingers by median; ring and little fingers by ulnar

(continued on following page)

Extrinsic Hand Extensors

Dorsal Wrist/Compartment/ Muscle(s)	Nerve	Test
1 *Abductor pollicis longus* *Extensor pollicis brevis*	R R	With all fingers extended, patient abducts thumb, keeping it in the plane of the other fingers.
2 *Extensor carpi radialis longus* *Extensor carpi radialis brevis*	R R	Clenching a fist, the patient extends at the wrist against resistance. Tendons palpable over dorsoradial wrist.
3 *Extensor pollicis longus*	R	Hand palm-down on table, patient lifts thumb straight up.
4 *Extensor digitorum communis* *Extensor indicis proprius*	R R	Extension simultaneously of 2nd through 5th fingers, examiner noting MCP extension. Test EIP separately by extension of index finger from a clenched fist, noting MCP extension.
5 *Extensor digiti minimi*	R	After making a fist, patient extends little finger. Examiner notes extension at MCP joint.
6 *Extensor carpi ulnaris*	R	Patient extends wrist and deviates it to the ulnar side. Tendon palpable over dorsal wrist distal to ulnar head.

HAND MOTOR EXAM *(cont.)*

Intrinsic Hand Muscles

Group	Muscle(s)	Nerve	Test
Thenar	*Abductor pollicis brevis*	M	Patient touches thumb to little finger keeping nails parallel.
	Opponens pollicis	M	
	Flexor pollicis brevis	M, U*	
	Adductor pollicis	U	Patient forcibly holds paper between thumb and radial side of the index proximal phalanx.
	Interosseous	U	Holding hand palm down, patient spreads fingers.
	Lumbricals	M, U†	
Hypothenar	*Abductor digiti minimi*	U	Holding hand palm down, and starting with fingers pressed together, the patient moves the little finger away from the others.
	Flexor digiti minimi	U	
	Opponens digiti minimi	U	

*Shared by median and ulnar
†Index and middle by median; ring and little fingers by ulnar

HAND MUSCLES BY NERVE INNERVATION

Median

Flexor carpi radialis
Palmaris longus
Flexor digitorum superficialis
Flexor digitorum profundus
   (thumb, index, and usually
   long fingers)
Flexor pollicis longus
Abductor pollicis brevis
Flexor pollicis brevis (shared
   with ulnar)
Opponens pollicis
Lumbricals (index and long
   fingers)

Radial

Extensor carpi radialis longus
   and *brevis*

Extensor digitorum communis
Extensor digiti minimi
Extensor carpi ulnaris
Abductor pollicis longus
Extensor pollicis longus and *brevis*
Extensor indicis proprius

Ulnar

Flexor carpi ulnaris
Flexor digitorum profundus (ring,
   little, and sometimes long fingers)
Adductor pollicis
Flexor pollicis brevis (shared with
   median)
Abductor, opponens, and *flexor digiti
   minimi*
Lumbricals (little and ring fingers)
   Interossei

HAND SENSORY NERVE INNERVATION

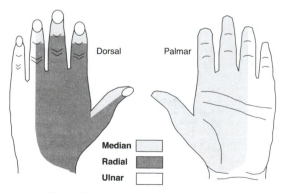

Figure 2–3   Muscle sensory nerve innervation.

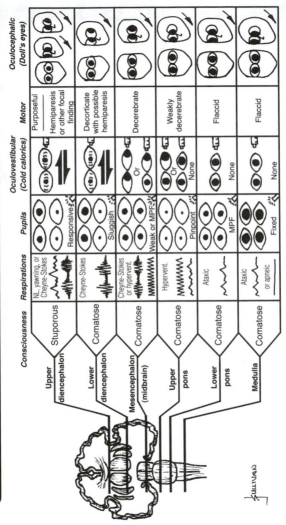

Figure 2–4 Coma: correlating exam findings with level of brain dysfunction.

*Dysconjugate response indicates structural brainstem lesion. MPF = mid-position fixed.

§Doll's-eye testing contraindicated in patients with suspected cervical spine injury.

NIH STROKE SCALE

Exam Variable	Score
1. Level of consciousness	
1a. Alert	0
Not alert, but arousable by minor stimulation	1
Not alert, requires repeated stimulation to attend	2
Coma or responds only with reflex motor or autonomic effects	3
1b. Ask the patient the month and their age	
Answers both correctly	0
Answers one correctly	1
Answers both incorrectly	2
1c. Ask the patient to open/close eyes AND grip/release non-paretic hand	
Performs both tasks correctly	0
Performs one task correctly	1
Performs neither correctly	2
2. Assess horizontal gaze	
Normal	0
Partial gaze palsy (one or both eyes)	1
Complete gaze palsy or forced deviation	2
3. Visual field testing	
No visual loss	0
Partial hemianopia	1
Complete hemianopia	2
Bilateral hemianopia (including cortical blindness)	3
4. Facial palsy testing (ask pt to show teeth, raise eyebrows, and close eyes)	
Normal symmetrical movement	0
Minor paralysis (flattened nasolabial fold, asymmetry on smiling)	1
Partial paralysis (near or total paralysis of lower face)	2
Complete paralysis (absence of upper and lower facial movement)	3

(continued on following page)

NIH STROKE SCALE *(cont.)*

5. Arm motor function (palms down with scoring of right and left individually)

No drift (limb maintained at 90° [standing] or 45° [sitting] for 10sec)	0
Drift <10sec, but not hitting bed or other support	1
Some effort against gravity, but cannot get to or maintain elevation	2
No effort against gravity	3
No movement	4

6. Leg motor function (score right and left individually)

No drift (limb maintained at 30° for 5sec)	0
Drift <5sec, but not hitting bed	1
Some effort against gravity, but cannot get to or maintain elevation	2
No effort against gravity	3
No movement	4

7. Limb ataxia (finger to nose and heel to shin performed bilaterally)

Absent	0
Present in one limb	1
Present in two limbs	2

8. Sensory loss (pinprick testing of arms, legs, trunk, and face with bilateral comparison)

Normal; no sensory loss	0
Mild to moderate; dullness or loss of pain, but aware of touch	1
Severe to total loss; no pain and no awareness to touch	2

9. Best language (assessed by describing picture, naming items, and reading sentences)

No aphasia	0
Mild to moderate aphasia; loss of fluency, without limitation of ideas	1
Severe aphasia; fragmented expression	2
Global aphasia (or mute); incomprehensible speech	3

10. Dysarthria (assessment of articulation through reading or repeating words)

(continued on following page)

Normal	0
Mild to moderate slurring	1
Severe slurring as to be unintelligible	2
Intubated or other physical barrier	3

11. Extinction and inattention (formerly neglect)

No abnormality	0
Inattention or extinction to bilateral simultaneous stimulation in one of the sensory modalities	1
Profound hemi-inattention; orients to one side of space only	2

Interpretation of Score

Total possible range = 0-42
0-5 = minor stroke
6-13 = moderate stroke
≥14 = major stroke

CLINICALLY USEFUL FORMULAE

Mean arterial (or pulmonary) pressure =
Diastolic pressure + (1/3 × pulse pressure)
Pressure in mm Hg = pressure in cm H_2O/1.36

Arterial blood O_2 content (CaO_2) =
(paO_2 × .003) + (1.34 × Hb in g × arterial blood Hb O_2 sat %);
Normal = 18-20ml/dl

Venous blood O_2 content (CvO_2) =
(pvO_2 × .003) + (1.34 × Hb in g × venous blood Hb O_2 sat %);
Normal = 13-16ml/dl

Arteriovenous O_2 difference ($avDO_2$) =
(CaO_2) − (CvO_2) *Normal* = 4-5ml/dl

O_2 delivery index (DO_2I) =
CaO_2 × cardiac index × 10; *Normal* = 500 - 600ml/min-m²

Shunt % =
(CcO_2 − CaO_2)/(CcO_2 − CvO_2)
CcO_2 = Hb in gm × 1.34 + (Alveolar pO_2 × .003); *Normal* < 10%;
Considerable disease = 20%-29%; *Life threatening* > 30%

Alveolar pO_2 =
[FIO_2 × (ambient atmospheric pressure* − 47)] − (1.2 × $paCO_2$)
* 760torr at sea level

Alveolar - Arterial O_2 difference or "A-a gradient" or $p(A-a)O_2$ =
Alveolar pO_2 − paO_2; *Normal* <10torr

Calculated osmolality =
2 [Na^+] + BUN/2.8 + glucose/18 + ethanol/4.6 + methanol/3.2 +
ethylene glycol/6.4
Normal = ~285

Osmolal gap =
measured osmolality − calculated osmolality; normal = 2 ± 6

Free water deficit
Total free water deficit (liters) =
(Serum [Na^+]/140) × (Weight [kg] × 0.6)

Centigrade-to-Fahrenheit temperature conversion °F =
(°C × 1.8) + 32

(continued on following page)

Fahrenheit-to-centigrade temperature conversion $°C =$
$(°F - 32)/1.8$

Pressure in mm Hg =
pressure in cm $H_2O/1.36$

Acid-base formulae: see p. 71.

Renal failure/creatinine clearance formulae: see p. 72.

ATLS PRIMARY AND SECONDARY SURVEYS

Primary

A **A**irway, maintain cervical spine control
B **B**reathing and ventilation
C **C**irculation with hemorrhage control
D **D**isability, neurologic status
E **E**xpose/**E**nvironmental control: undress completely, prevent hypothermia
G **G**astric decompression

Secondary

- Complete head-to-toe evaluation; repeat vital signs; neurologic exam, including Glasgow Coma Scale
- Special procedures: peritoneal lavage, radiologic evaluation, laboratory studies, IV line placement
- "Tubes and fingers in every orifice"
- History: **AMPLE** – **A**llergies, **M**edications currently taken, **P**ast illnesses, **L**ast meal, **E**vents/**E**nvironment related to injury

CLASSIFICATION OF HEMORRHAGIC SHOCK

Class I ≤15% blood loss: minimal clinical symptoms
Class II 15%-30% blood loss (750-1500cc): tachycardia, narrow pulse pressure, anxiety, minimal change in urine output
Class III 30%-40% blood loss (2000cc): tachycardia, tachypnea, pale, diaphoretic, hypotensive
Class IV >40% blood loss: immediately life-threatening with marked tachycardia/tachypnea, significant hypotension, no urine output, mental status changes (>50% blood loss results in LOC + absent vital signs).

REVISED ADULT TRAUMA SCORE

Criterion	Score	Criterion	Score
Respiratory Rate		*Survival Probability by Trauma Score**	
10-24	**4**	12	0.995
25-35	**3**	11	0.969
36·≥	**2**	10	0.879
1-9	**1**	9	0.766
0	**0**	8	0.667
		7	0.636
Systolic Blood Pressure		6	0.63
90·≥	**4**	5	0.455
76-89	**3**	4	0.333
50-75	**2**	3	0.333
1-49	**1**	2	0.286
0 (no pulse)	**0**	1	0.25
		0	0.037
Glasgow Coma Scale (see page xxx)			
Coma scale 13-15	**4**	*Survival Probability by Pediatric Trauma Score (see below)†*	
Coma scale 9-12	**3**	12	1.00
Coma scale 6-8	**2**	10	1.00
Coma scale 4-5	**1**	8	0.98
Coma scale 3	**0**	6	0.92
		4	0.68
		2	0.60
		0	0.26
		−2	0.08
		−4	0.00

*Source: *J Trauma* 1989; 29:623.
†Source: *J Pediatr Surg* 1987; 22:14.

PEDIATRIC TRAUMA SCORE

*Patients with a total score of <8 should be triaged to a Pediatric Trauma Center.**

Score	+2	1	−1
Weight	>20kg	10–20kg	<10kg
Airway	Normal	Oral or nasal airway	Intubation or cricothyroidotomy
Blood pressure	>90 mm Hg	50–90mm Hg	<50mm Hg
Level of con- sciousness	Awake and alert	Obtunded or any LOC	Comatose
Open wound	None	Minor	Major or penetrating
Fractures	None	Single simple	Open or multiple

*For survival by Pediatric Trauma Score, see above.

ADULT GLASGOW COMA SCALE

Criterion	Score
Eye-Opening Response	
Spontaneous – already open with blinking	4
To speech – not necessary to request eye opening	3
To pain – stimulus should not be to the face	2
None – make note if eyes are swollen shut	1
Verbal Response	
Oriented – knows name, age, etc.	5
Confused conversation – still answers questions	4
Inappropriate words – speech exclamatory or random	3
Incomprehensible sounds, but no partial respiratory obstruction	2
None – make note if patient is intubated	1
Best Upper Limb Motor Response (Pressure Applied to Nailbed)	
Obeys – moves limb to command; pain is not required	6
Localizes – change location of painful stimulus, limb follows	5
Withdraws – pulls away from painful stimulus	4
Abnormal flexion – decorticate posturing	3
Extensor response – decerebrate posturing	2
No response	1

PEDIATRIC (INFANT) COMA SCALE

	Score	Response		Score	Response
Eye opening	4	Spontaneous	*Motor response*	6	Spontaneous movement
	3	To speech or sound		5	Localizes pain
	2	To painful stimuli		4	Withdraws in response to pain
	1	None			
Verbal response	5	Coos, babbles		3	Flexes – decorticate
	4	Irritable cry, consolable		2	Extends – decerebrate
	3	Cries in response to pain		1	None
	2	Moans in response to pain			
	1	None			

CERVICAL SPINE INJURIES: STABLE AND UNSTABLE

Flexion

Wedge fx	*Stable*
Clay-shoveler's fx	*Stable*
Subluxation	*Potentially unstable*
Bilateral facet dislocation	*Unstable*
Flexion teardrop	*Unstable*
Atlanto-occipital dislocation	*Unstable*
Anterior atlantoaxial dislocation ± fx	*Unstable*
Odontoid fx + lateral displacement	*Unstable*
Fx of transverse process	*Stable*

Extension

Posterior neural arch fx, C1	*Stable*
Hangman's fx, C2	*Unstable*
Extension teardrop fx	*Unstable in extension; stable in flexion*
Posterior atlantoaxial dislocation ± fx	*Unstable*

Vertical Compression

Burst fx	*Stable*
Jefferson fx, C1	*Unstable*
Fx of articular pillar and vertebral body	*Stable*

Rotation

Unilateral facet dislocation	*Stable*
Rotary atlantoaxial dislocation	*Unstable*

NEXUS CRITERIA FOR SPINE INJURY

Cervical spine imaging indicated in patients with blunt trauma unless they meet all five criteria.

1. No posterior midline cervical spine tenderness, with palpation from nuchal ridge to 1st thoracic vertebra
2. No evidence of intoxication
3. A normal level of alertness (defined as GCS >14; orientation to person, place, time, and events; ability to remember three objects at 5min; and appropriate response to **external** stimulation)
4. No focal neurologic deficit
5. No painful distracting injuries (including but not limited to long-bone fractures, visceral injuries necessitating surgical consultation, large lacerations, degloving injuries, crush injuries, or large burns)

Adapted from: *N Engl J Med* 2000; 343:94.

CERVICAL SPINE RADIOLOGIC PARAMETERS

In Lateral View

Atlanto-dental interval = distance from anterior aspect of odontoid to posterior aspect of C1 (**a**). Normal = 0-3mm (children, 0-4.5mm). In adults, 3-7mm indicates rupture of transverse ligament; >7mm indicates rupture of alar and apical dentate ligaments.

If the anterior height of any vertebral body (**b1**) is greater by more than 3mm than the posterior height (**b2**), a vertebral body fracture is likely.

Soft tissue from anterior aspect of each vertebral body to tracheal air space should measure not more than the following:

- At C1 (**c**), 10mm.
- At the bottom of C2 (**d**), 5mm.
- At the bottom of C3 (**e**), 7mm.
- From the bottom of C5 to the bottom of C7 (**f**), 20mm.

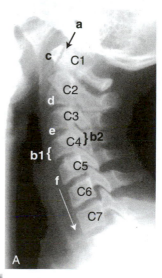

In AP Odontoid View

In AP view, sum of overhang of both facets of C1 on C2 >7mm = rupture of transverse ligament (**g**).

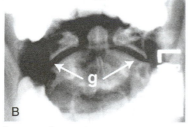

Concept and research courtesy of Steve Yucht, M.D.

OTTAWA ANKLE RULES

An ankle radiograph series is required only if there is any pain in the malleolar zone and any of these findings is present:

1. Bone tenderness at posterior edge or tip of lateral malleolus.
2. Bone tenderness at posterior edge or tip of medial malleolus.
3. Inability to bear weight both immediately and in the ED.

A foot radiographic series is required only if there is any pain in the midfoot zone and any of these findings is present:

1. Bone tenderness at base of the fifth metatarsal.
2. Bone tenderness at the navicular.
3. Inability to bear weight both immediately and in the ED.

Source: JAMA 1993; 269:827–832.

PITTSBURGH KNEE RULES

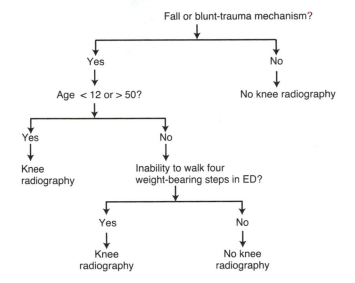

RABIES: INDICATIONS FOR PROPHYLAXIS *(SEE P. 133 FOR TREATMENT)*

Geographic Area	Animals	Treatment Recommendation	
		Bite	*Non-Bite Contact[§]*
Group 1: rabies endemic or suspected in species involved in the exposure	Bats, skunks, foxes; mongooses in Puerto Rico; dogs in most developing countries and in the U.S. along Mexican border (3%–80% rabid)	*Treat**	*Treat**
Group 2: rabies not endemic in species involved in the exposure, but endemic in other terrestrial animals in area	Most wild carnivores (wolves, bobcats, bears) and groundhogs (2%–20% rabid)	*Treat**	*Treat* or consult†*
	Dogs and cats (0.1%–2% rabid)	*Observe¶ or consult†*	*Observe¶ or consult†*
	Rodents and lagomorphs except groundhogs (about 0.01% rabid)	*Consult† or do not treat*	*Do not treat*
Group 3: rabies not endemic in species involved in the exposure or in other terrestrial animals in area	Dogs, cats, many wild terrestrial animals in Washington, Idaho, Utah, Nevada, Colorado (0.01%–0.1% rabid)	*Consult† or do not treat*	*Consult† or do not treat*

[§]Rabies develops in 5%–60% if bitten, 0.1%–0.2% if scratched or licked in open wound or mucous membrane.
*Treat = treatment with rabies immune globulin (RIG) and rabies vaccine – see p. xxx for treatment details.
†Consult = with state/local health dept. If rabies risk low and animal's brain available, Rx sometimes delayed up to 48h.
¶Observe = After bite from domestic dog/cat, confine animal for 10d; if signs of rabies occur, treat immediately. After bite from stray or unwanted dog/cat, animal should be killed and head shipped to qualified lab for exam.

By permission of *N Engl J Med* 1993; 329:1635.

ADULT BURN SURFACE AREA

"Rule of nines"

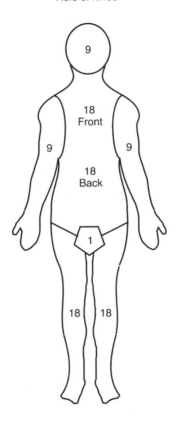

PEDIATRIC BURN SURFACE AREA

Body Area	Age in years			
	0–1	1–4	4–9	10–15
Head	19	17	13	10
Neck	2	2	2	2
Chest or back (each)	13	13	13	13
Buttock (each)	2.5	2.5	2.5	2.5
Genitalia	1	1	1	1
Upper arm (each)	4	4	4	4
Lower arm (each)	3	3	3	3
Hand (each)	2.5	2.5	2.5	2.5
Thigh (each)	5.5	6.5	8.5	8.5
Lower leg (each)	5	5	5	6
Foot (each)	3.5	3.5	3.5	3.5

INDICATIONS FOR ADMISSION: ADULTS AND CHILDREN

- Partial thickness >20% or full thickness >10%.
- Burns of hands, face, eyes, ears, feet, or perineum.
- Inhalation injury, electrical burns, or associated serious trauma.
- High-risk patient, i.e., diabetes, obesity, liver disease, suspected child abuse.

FLUID MANAGEMENT ADULTS AND CHILDREN

Ringer's lactate 2-4ml/kg/% of body surface area over the first 24h with half over the first 8h and the remainder over the ensuing 16h, calculated from the time the burn is sustained. Add maintenance fluids for infants. This formula is meant as a guide – fluid management should be adjusted in accordance with clinical signs.

TETANUS PROPHYLAXIS

Adequacy of tetanus immunization should be ascertained, and toxoid and immune globulin administered when indicated (p. 46).

TETANUS WOUND PROPHYLAXIS

Number of Previous TD Doses	Tetanus-Prone Wounds (See #4 Below)		Non–Tetanus-Prone Wounds	
	Toxoid	*TIG*	*Toxoid*	*TIG*
Not known	Yes	Yes	Yes	No
0-1	Yes	Yes	Yes	No
2	Yes	No*	Yes	No
3·≥	No#	No	No†	No

*Yes if wound more than 24 hours old.
#Yes if more than 5 years since last dose.
†Yes if more than 10 years since last dose.

Note:

1. For children less than 7y.o., diphtheria-tetanus-pertussis (DPT) is pre-ferred unless pertussis is contraindicated; all others should receive diphtheria-tetanus (TD).
2. TIG = tetanus immune globulin. Dose is 250-500U IM for both children and adults.
3. When TIG and TD are given concurrently, use separate syringes and inject at separate sites.
4. Tetanus-prone wounds are suggested by:
   - More than 12 hours since injury
   - Blunt mechanism of injury
   - Signs of infection present
   - Devitalized or ischemic tissue present
   - Contaminants – soil, feces, saliva – in wound

CT GRADING OF SOLID ORGAN INJURIES

Spleen

Grade	Injury
I	Subcapsular hematoma <10% of surface area or laceration <1cm deep
II	Subcapsular hematoma 10%-50% of surface area or laceration 1-3cm deep
III	Subcapsular hematoma >50% of surface area or expanding, intraparenchymal hematoma >5cm or expanding, or laceration >3cm deep
IV	Laceration involving segmental or hilar vessels with >25% devascularization or actively bleeding intra-parenchymal hematoma
V	Completely shattered or devascularized spleen

Liver

Grade	Injury
I	Subcapsular hematoma <10% of surface area or laceration <1cm deep
II	Subcapsular hematoma 10%–50% of surface area or laceration 1-3cm deep but <10cm long
III	Subcapsular hematoma >50% of surface area or expanding, or laceration >3cm deep
IV	Parenchymal disruption involving 25%-75% of hepatic lobe or 1-4 Couinaud's segments in a single lobe
V	Parenchymal disruption >75% of lobe or >3 Couinaud's segments or juxtahepatic venous injuries (retro-hepatic vena cava or hepatic veins)
VI	Hepatic avulsion

Kidney

Grade	Injury
I	Contusions: hematuria with normal urological studies or subcapsular, non-expanding hematoma without parenchymal laceration
II	Non-expanding subcapsular hematoma, perirenal hematoma confined to retroperitoneum, or laceration <1cm depth of renal cortex

(continued on following page)

CT GRADING OF SOLID ORGAN INJURIES *(cont.)*

Grade	Injury
III	Laceration >1cm depth of renal cortex without collecting system rupture or urinary extravasation
IV	Laceration of parenchyma extending through cortex, medulla, and collecting system or involving main renal vasculature (artery or vein) with contained hemorrhage
V	Completely shattered kidney or avulsion through renal hilum with complete devascularization

Adapted from: *American Association for the Surgery of Trauma.*

CHAPTER 4 | *TOXICOLOGY*

GENERAL PROTOCOL FOR INGESTIONS

I. Gastrointestinal decontamination
   A. Routine *gastric emptying* is not recommended. It can be considered when (1) ingestion of a potentially fatal poison has occurred, and (2) it can be performed soon after ingestion. *Syrup of Ipecac* (SOI) can be given when (1) there is no contraindication to its use, (2) alternative therapy is not available or effective, or (3) when pre-hospital delays of >1h are anticipated. SOI dosing is as follows: *Ambulatory children < 12y.o.:* 15ml po. *Child >12y.o.-adult:* 30ml po. Ideally, SOI should be given within 30min of ingestion and in consultation with a poison control center/medical toxicologist. SOI is contraindicated after ingestion of an agent that has CNS/cardiovascular toxicity, is corrosive, or if gag reflex is absent. *Gastric lavage* should be carried out within 60min of exposure. Pre-lavage intubation should be considered when there is risk of aspiration. Late gastric lavage can be considered in patients who are critically ill, have ingested a massive amount of a life-threatening agent, or have ingested substances that are sustained-release, poorly digested, or cause pylorospasm.
   B. *Activated charcoal* 0.5-1g/kg should be considered up to 1h after a potentially toxic ingestion. Avoid in patients who have ingested hydrocarbons or corrosive substances.
   C. *Whole bowel irrigation using polyethylene glycol-containing solutions* is an option for (1) potentially toxic ingestions of substances not bound to activated charcoal (iron, lithium, other metals); (2) sustained-release or enteric-coated drugs; (3) ingested packets of illicit drugs; or (4) massive ingestions. *Child:* 20-40ml/kg/h. *Adult:* 1-2 liters/h. Administer until rectal effluent is clear. Contraindicated if ileus present or there is risk of aspiration.
   D. *Multiple dose activated charcoal (MDAC)* 0.5g/kg Q 2-4h with one dose of cathartic/day can be considered for a patient who has ingested a life-threatening amount of carbamazepine, dapsone, phenobarbital, quinine, theophylline, amatoxin (mushroom), or colchicine. MDAC for patients with salicylate, phenytoin, digoxin/

(continued on following page)

GENERAL PROTOCOL FOR INGESTIONS *(cont.)*

digitoxin, amitriptyline, propoxyphene, disopyramide, atenolol, nadolol, sotalol, phenylbutazone, or piroxicam poisoning is controversial. Contraindicated if ileus present.

E. *Cathartics* should be considered with the first dose of activated charcoal, and QD if MDAC is used. *Sorbitol* 0.5-1g/kg is most effective but must not be given if an ileus is present, if there risk of aspiration, or if age <12 mo.

II. Observation

All patients with alleged ingestion should be closely observed for at least 6h on a cardiac monitor. When in doubt as to the nature of the ingestion, administer activated charcoal and observe. Remember: a negative drug screen does not rule out ingestion of a toxic agent. If exposure to the substances listed in Toxic Time Bombs (see p. 54) occurs, prolonged observation (18-24h) should be considered.

PROTOCOL FOR CUTANEOUS DECONTAMINATION

Hospital personnel must don appropriate protective equipment prior to patient decontamination. Do outdoors if possible.

(1) Eye and wound irrigation should receive priority. Irrigate continuously with normal saline or lactated Ringer's solution.

(2) Clothing should be removed as soon as possible. Particulate or radioactive matter should be removed by careful roll-down of clothing. Any remaining particulate matter should be brushed away prior to showering.

(3) Whole body decontamination should begin with the hands, face, and head, which are generally the most heavily contaminated areas. Head-back position is desirable.

(4) Most chemicals are readily removed with copious amounts of tepid water (exception: elemental metals explode with water contact), and special decontamination solutions are rarely necessary. Attempting to obtain such decontamination often delays decontamination.

(5) A mild soap, shampoo, or detergent may be necessary for nonpolar, water-insoluble substances.

(6) In children, the focus should be on decontamination of parent-child pairs using a high-volume, low pressure warm water delivery system that allows both supervision and thermoregulation.

(7) 3-5min of showering is recommended, although 15min may be required for concentrated, strongly alkaline materials or oily, adherent

(continued on following page)

substances. The use of abrasives, such as corn meal or scrub brushes, is generally not advised—abrading the skin may increase toxin absorption.

(8) Specific cutaneous decontamination solutions/antidotes:

- (a) Phenol: isopropanol, polyethylene glycol solutions.
- (b) Phosphorus: ignites on contact with air. Keep covered with oil. Wood's lamp detects.
- (c) Hydrofluoric acid: apply topically 2.5-10% calcium gluconate gel until pain relief.
  1. For hand injuries: infuse calcium gluconate 10% 10ml in 40ml D₅W via radial artery over 4h while on cardiac monitor. Consult hand surgeon.
  2. All other areas: inject calcium gluconate 10% 0.5ml/sq cm of involved tissue.
  3. For systemic fluoride poisoning: *Child:* 0.2-0.3ml/kg IV. *Adult:* 10-30ml calcium gluconate IV.
- (d) Water-reative metals (sodium, potassium, lithium): cover with mineral oil, remove with forceps.
- (e) Cyanoacrylates: acetone (skin), mineral oil, or saline-soaked gauze pads (eyes).
- (f) Tar: Neosporin, Tween 80, Vaseline, Desolvit, mayonnaise. Tar should be allowed to cool prior to removal—mechanical removal can increase tissue destruction and result in hair follicle loss.

PROTOCOL FOR TRICYCLIC ANTIDEPRESSANT INGESTIONS

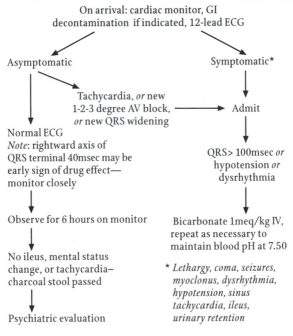

On arrival: cardiac monitor, GI decontamination if indicated, 12-lead ECG

Asymptomatic

Symptomatic*

Tachycardia, *or* new 1-2-3 degree AV block, *or* new QRS widening

Admit

Normal ECG
Note: rightward axis of QRS terminal 40msec may be early sign of drug effect—monitor closely

QRS> 100msec *or* hypotension *or* dysrhythmia

Observe for 6 hours on monitor

Bicarbonate 1meq/kg IV, repeat as necessary to maintain blood pH at 7.50

No ileus, mental status change, or tachycardia–charcoal stool passed

* *Lethargy, coma, seizures, myoclonus, dysrhythmia, hypotension, sinus tachycardia, ileus, urinary retention*

Psychiatric evaluation

Osmolality Formula

Calculated osmolality = 2Na + BUN/2.8 + Glucose/18
Normal = 285–295mOsm/kg

If measured osmolality (by freezing point depression) is more than 10 greater than calculated osmolality, unmeasured osmoles should be presumed to be present. However, a normal "gap" does not rule out the presence of toxic alcohols.

Osmol Ratios: to calculate contribution to measured osmolality in mOsm/kg, divide concentration in mg/dl by these numbers:

Ethylene glycol	*Isopropanol*	*Ethanol*	*Methanol*
6.2	6.0	4.6	3.2

Acetaminophen Overdose Nomogram

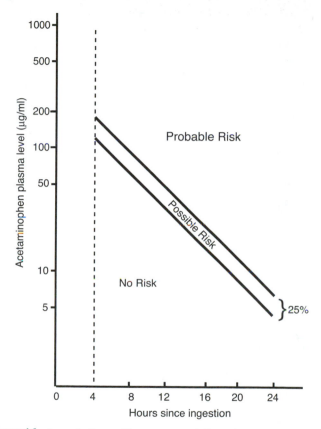

Figure 4-1 For evaluating need for treatment with N-acetylcysteine (NAC), based on time since a single, acute ingestion and plasma concentration on presentation. Treatment should be considered when levels fall above the area of "no risk." Determinations before 4 hours may not represent peak levels. If coingestants or extended-release acetaminophen has been ingested, obtain 4h and 8h levels; if either is above "no-risk," NAC is recommended. (Reproduced with permission, *Arch Intern Med* 1981; 141:380–385. Copyright AMA.)

Toxic Time Bombs

TOXINS FOR WHICH PROLONGED MONITORING SHOULD BE CONSIDERED FOLLOWING EXPOSURE

Toxin	Delayed Toxicity Manifestation
Acrylonitrile, acetonitrile, propionitrile	Cyanide toxicity
Aniline	Methemoglobinemia
Antidiarrheals: diphenoxylate/ loperamide (*Lomotil®, Imodium®*)	CNS, respiratory depression
Arsine	Hemolysis
Benzene	Bone marrow suppression and leukemia
Botulism	Neuroparalysis, respiratory depression
Calcium channel blockers, sustained-release	Cardiovascular collapse
Cadmium	Pneumonitis
Castor bean (ricin)	Gastrointestinal, multisystem organ failure
Chemotherapeutics	Bone marrow suppression, multisystem organ failure
Chlorine	Pulmonary edema (if symptomatic)
Colchicine	Multisystem organ failure
Coral snake/Mojave rattlesnake	Neurologic toxicity
Cyanogenic plants	Cyanide toxicity
Dapsone	Methemoglobinemia, hemolysis
Ethylene glycol	CNS, cardiopulmonary, renal toxicity; acidosis
Ethylene oxide	Pulmonary edema and neurotoxicity
Hypoglycemics (sulfonylureas)	Hypoglycemia
Halogenated solvents (ingestion)	Hepatorenal toxicity
Hydrofluoric acid	Pulmonary edema, dermal burns, electrolyte disorders
Hydrogen sulfide	Pulmonary edema
MAO inhibitors	Cardiovascular collapse, seizures, hyperadrenergic state

Toxin	Delayed Toxicity Manifestation
Methadone	CNS, respiratory depression
Methanol	Neurologic (CNS, blindness), acid-base disturbance
Methyl bromide	Pulmonary edema
Methylene chloride	Carbon monoxide toxicity, dysrhythmias
Mushrooms	
Amanita phalloides	Hepatic necrosis
Gyromitra esculenta	Neuro/hepatic/methemoglobinemia
Nail primers with oxidants (nitroethane, paratoluidine)	Methemoglobinemia, skin/GI burns
Nitrogen oxides	Pulmonary edema, methemoglobinemia
Organophosphates (highly lipid soluble, or dermal exposure to nerve agents)	Cholinergic toxicity
Ozone (rare)	Pulmonary edema
Paraquat, diquat	Pulmonary fibrosis
Pennyroyal oil (not leaves)	Hepatotoxicity
Phenylbutazone	Cardiopulmonary, aplastic anemia
Phosgene	Pulmonary edema
Phosphine	Pulmonary edema
Podophyllin	Multisystem organ failure
Rodenticides	
Bromethalin	Uncoupled oxidative phosphorylation/neurotoxicity
Na monofluoroacetate (1080)	Shock, hypocalcemia, multisystem organ failure
Vacor	Hyperglycemia, autonomic neuropathy
Rosary pea (abrin)	Gastrointestinal/multisystem organ failure
Thioridazine/mesoridazine	Cardiac arrhythmias
TCAs in children (?)	Seizures, hypotension, arrhythmias
Zinc phosphide*	Pulmonary edema

*Indicates agent for which significant OD may be more easily ruled out than for other listed agents.

TOXIDROMES

Drug	Symptoms/Signs	Management Principles
Sympathomimetics (Cocaine, amphetamines)	Tachycardia, tachypnea, mydriasis, hyperthermia, altered mentation, coma, agitation, seizure, rhabdomyolysis.	Benzodiazepines IV for agitation, aggressive cooling, short-acting cardiovascular agents, benzodiazepines and barbiturates for seizures, measures to correct acidosis.
Anticholinergics (Antihistamines, over-the-counter sleep aids, antipsychotics, plants, and mushrooms)	Central: altered mentation, coma, agitation, seizure, hyperthermia. Peripheral: tachycardia, ileus, urinary retention, mydriasis, dry skin and mucous membranes, flushing.	Same as for sympathomimetics. Physostigmine only for intractable seizures or supraventricular tachycardia with hemodynamic instability. Dose: 0.5mg over 5min (child) or 1-2mg IV over 5min (adult).
Cholinergics (Organophosphates, carbamates)	Vomiting, diarrhea, salivation, lacrimation, bronchorrhea, miosis, fasciculations, paralysis.	Aggressive airway management and pulmonary toilet. For organophosphates/carbamates: atropine and pralidoxime – for dosing, see p. 58. Worsening of carbaryl OD reported with pralidoxime – avoid.
Opiates	CNS and respiratory depression, miosis, hypothermia. Meperidine may cause myoclonus/seizures, mydriasis. Propoxyphene may cause seizures and cardiac conduction blocks.	Naloxone – for dosing, see p. 60. Drugs that may necessitate higher doses of naloxone than other narcotics: methadone, pentazocine, propoxyphene, diphenoxylate, fentanyl.

ANTIDOTES TO SPECIFIC OVERDOSES

Overdose	Antidote	Initial Dose
Acetaminophen	N-acetylcysteine (*Mucomyst®*, *Acetadote®*)	*Child/adult:* 140mg/kg po initial dose, then 70mg/kg po Q 4h for 17 doses (see pp. 62-63).
Benzodiazepines	Flumazenil *See also pp. 196-197*	For reversal of CNS depression from overdose (*not for mixed ingestions or in pts who are chronically benzodiazepine dependent or in those with elevated ICP, agitation, or seizures*). *Child <20kg:* 0.01mg/kg IV/IM. *Child >20kg-adult:* 0.2mg IV/IM. May repeat initial dose Q 2-3min prn.
Beta-blockers	Glucagon *and/or* Atropine *and/or* Epinephrine *and/or* Calcium chloride 10% (for dosing, see below)	*Child:* 50μg/kg IV over 1min. *Adult:* 5-10mg IV over 1min. *Child/adult:* 0.01mg/kg IV. *Child/adult:* start 0.02μg/kg/min infusion, titrate to desired effect.
Botulism	Trivalent antitoxin	*Child/adult:* 1-2 vials.
Calcium channel blockers	Calcium chloride 10% *and/or* Glucagon *and/or* Beta-/alpha-adrenergic agonists *and/or*	*Child:* 20mg (0.2ml)/kg IV over 5min. *Adult:* 1g (10ml) IV over 5min. Give slowly while on a cardiac monitor. *Child:* 50μg/kg IV over 1min. *Adult:* 5-10mg IV over 1min. As needed.

(continued on following page)

57

ANTIDOTES TO SPECIFIC OVERDOSES (cont.)

Overdose	Antidote	Initial Dose
	Insulin/dextrose	*Child/adult:* Insulin 0.5U/kg/h with D10/D25 to euglycemia (evidence suggests supports cardiac output.)
Carbamates	Atropine	*Child:* 0.02mg/kg IV initial dose. *Adult:* 2mg IV initial dose. May require larger doses.
	Pralidoxime	Dosing as for organophosphates.
Carbamazepine	Sodium bicarbonate	*Same indications/dosing as for TCAs.*
Carbon monoxide	Hyperbaric oxygen	*Indications:* abnl mental status, COHb >25% or pregnant with COHb >10%-15%, syncope, cardiac ischemia, worsening sx despite normobaric oxygen.
Carbon disulfide	Pyridoxine (vitamin B6)	*Child/adult:* 70mg/kg IV over 15-30min (for seizures).
Cocaine	Sodium bicarbonate *and/or* Benzodiazepines	*Same indications/dosing as for TCAs.* Titrated by physician. Avoid β-blockers.
Coumarin compounds (warfarin) *For therapeutic OD, see p. 80*	Vitamin K1 *and/or* Fresh-frozen plasma	*Child <1y.o.:* 1mg in 20-50ml IV Q 4-8h. *Child >1y.o. -adult:* 5-10mg IV at 1mg/min. Dose variable.

Poison	Antidote	Dose
Cyanide *For smoke inhalation use only thiosulfate*	Amyl nitrite perles *and* Sodium nitrite 3% *and* Sodium thiosulfate 25% and 100% O2 mask	*Child/adult:* inhale 30sec/min in O₂ mask. *Child/adult:* 0.33ml/kg IV over 5min (max 10ml). *Adjust for anemia per manufacturer's insert.* *Child/adult:* 1.65ml/kg IV over 10min (max 50ml). *Child/adult:* concomitant with above.
Cyclic antidepressant	Sodium bicarbonate *See TCA protocol p. xxx*	*Child/adult:* if QRS >100 msec, hypotension, or arrhythmia: initial dose 1mEq/kg IV, then repeat boluses to maintain serum pH >7.5.
Digitalis	Digoxin-specific antibody fragments	*Child/adult:* dose in vials = *either:* (1) # pills × mg/pill × 1.17, or (2) (dig level in ng/ml × wt in kg)/100. If hemodynam. unstable, give 10-20 vials (40mg/vial) IV (*child/adult*).
Ethylene glycol	[(Ethanol 10% in D₅W *or* Fomepizole) *and* Pyridoxine *and* Thiamine]	*Child/adult:* 10ml/kg over 1h, then infuse 1ml/kg/h to target level of 100mg/dl. *Child/adult:* 15mg/kg IV over 30min. *Child/adult:* 50mg IV Q 6h. *Child:* 50mg IV QD. *Adult:* 100mg IV QD.
***Gyromitra esculenta* mushrooms**	Pyridoxine (vitamin B6)	*Child/adult:* 25mg/kg IV over 15–30min if neurologic symptoms present.
Heparin	Protamine sulfate	*Child/adult:* 1mg IV/100U heparin given.
Hydrogen sulfide	Sodium nitrite 3% (from cyanide kit)	*Child/adult:* 0.33ml/kg IV over 5min. Adjust for anemia per manufacturer's insert.

(continued on following page)

ANTIDOTES TO SPECIFIC OVERDOSES (cont.)

Overdose	Antidote	Initial Dose
Iron	Deferoxamine	*Child/adult:* for prolonged GI sx, lethargy, level >500mg/dl: 15mg/kg/h infusion.
Isoniazid	Pyridoxine (vitamin B6)	*Child:* 70mg/kg IV. *Adult:* 1mg IV for each mg of INH ingested; max 5g.
Methanol	[(Ethanol 10% in D_5W *or* Fomepizole) *and* Leucovorin]	*Child/adult:* 10ml/kg over 1h, then infuse 1ml/kg/h to target level of 100mg/dl. *Child/adult:* 15mg/kg IV over 30min. *Child/adult:* 1-2mg/kg IV Q 4-6h.
Methemoglobinemia	Methylene blue	*Child/adult:* for symptoms or if MetHg >30%: 1-2mg/kg.
Norpropoxyphene	Sodium bicarbonate	*Same indications/dosing as for TCAs.*
Opiates	Naloxone	*Child <20kg:* 0.1mg/kg IV. *Child >20kg to adult:* 0.4mg (0.05mg if opioid dependent) IV. Repeat to max 10mg. *Infusion:* give $^2/_3$ of that initially needed to awaken patient per hour IV.
Organophosphates	Atropine *and* Pralidoxime	*Child:* 0.02mg/kg/dose IV. *Adult:* 2mg/dose IV. *Repeat as necessary to dry lung secretions.* *Child:* 25-40mg/kg IV over 10min, max 1g; then 10-20mg/kg/h infusion. *Adult:* 1g IV over 10min, then 500mg/h infusion.

Phenothiazines *(Dystonic reaction only)*	Diphenhydramine *or* Benztropine mesylate	*Child:* 1-2mg/kg IV slowly. *Adult:* 25-50mg IM/IV. *Adult (only):* 1-2mg IM/IV.
Quinidine/quinine	Sodium bicarbonate	*Same dosing/indications as for TCAs.*
Salicylates	Sodium bicarbonate	If serum pH <7.40, give 1mEq/kg bolus. In all cases, give bicarb as needed to keep blood pH 7.45-7.50, urine pH 7.5-8.0.
Sulfonylureas	Octreotide	*Child:* 1-1.25μg/kg SC Q 6h. *Adult:* 50μg SC Q 6h.
Tricyclic antide-pressants Type IA/ IC antiarrhythmics	Sodium bicarbonate *See TCA protocol p. 52*	*Child/adult:* if QRS >100msec, hypotension, or arrhythmia: initial dose 1mEq/kg IV, then repeat boluses to maintain serum pH >7.5.
Warfarin *For therapeutic OD, see p. 80*	Vitamin K1 *and/or*	*Child <1y.o.:* 1mg in 20-50ml IV Q 4-8h. *Child >1y.o. to adult:* 5-10mg IV at 1mg/min.
	Fresh-frozen plasma	Dose variable.

N-ACETYLCYSTEINE (MUCOMYST® OR ACETADOTE®) TREATMENT OF ACETAMINOPHEN INGESTION

Mucomyst® is the traditional form of N-acetylcysteine (NAC) used for po treatment or constituted by hospital pharmacists for IV administration. Acetadote® is a recently approved IV-ready formulation of NAC. In most situations, they are therapeutically equivalent.

The oral dosing for both *child/adult* of NAC is 140mg/kg po, then 70mg/kg po Q 4h for 17 doses. It is most effective when given within 8h of ingestion but is beneficial later.

IV NAC is equally but not more effective than the oral route in uncomplicated cases. However, patients with hepatotoxicity (transaminases >1000) may benefit from IV NAC. As there is considerable risk of serious adverse reactions with the IV route (up to 18% may develop anaphylactoid reactions), the oral route is generally preferred. We consider the FDA-approved IV formulation (Acetadote®) therapeutically equivalent to oral NAC constituted for IV administration.

IV NAC should be considered when there is evidence of significant hepatic necrosis (AST or ALT >1000) or when po administration is likely to be unsuccessful, e.g., with intractable emesis, when the patient must be NPO, or with ileus, caustic esophageal burns, or when the patient is pregnant.

Administration of Intravenous NAC

1. *Precautions:* patients with asthma should be given only the IV route after careful consideration of risks/benefits. *Monitoring:* monitor patients for signs of anaphylactoid reactions/fever. Discuss risks/ benefits of IV administration. Anaphylactoid reactions are dose- and possibly administration rate-related and occur most commonly during loading. They include hypotension, rash, flushing, chest pain, tachycardia, bronchospasm, and angioedema. *Treatment:* stop infusion, give antihistamines or, for severe cases, epinephrine. May resume after 1h at slower rate or convert to po dosing.
2. Treatment can be changed to po from IV if GI intolerance resolves.
3. With hepatotoxicity, continue NAC IV until transaminases <1000.
4. **Oral NAC (Mucomyst®) for IV treatment:** *Child/adult:* Dilute all doses of Mucomyst® 20% (20g/100ml) sltn 1 part with 5 parts D5W to make an approximately 3% (3g/100ml = 30mg/ml) sltn, and give IV over 1h. (More rapid rates may cause serious reactions.) The **loading dose** is 140mg/kg. (*Example:* A 50kg patient requires a loading dose of 7g or 35ml of 20% Mucomyst®. Mix the 35ml in 175ml of D5W for a total

(continued on following page)

volume of 210ml and give IV over 1h.) Then give subsequent **intermittent doses** of 70mg/kg IV over 1h Q 4h.

5. **Acetadote® for IV treatment**: *Child:* Mix 50ml of Acetadote® (20% sltn [20g/100ml] in 30ml/vial) with 200ml of D_5W (remove 50ml from a 250ml bag of D_5W) to obtain a 4% (4g/100ml = 40mg/ml) concentration. (This provides enough NAC for a complete course for children ≤33 kg.) Give a **loading dose** of 150mg/kg (3.75ml/kg) IV over 1h, then give a **second infusion** of 50mg/kg (1.25ml/kg) IV over 4h (0.31ml/kg/h), then give a **third infusion** of 100mg/kg (2.5ml/kg) IV over 16h (0.16ml/kg/h). *Adult:* Use the FDA-approved IV 20h protocol. We advise giving the loading dose over 1h rather than the 15min recommended by the package insert. Give a **loading dose** of 150mg/kg in 200ml of D_5W IV over 1h, then give a **second infusion** of 50mg/kg diluted in 500ml of D_5W IV over 4h, then give a **third infusion** of 100mg/kg in 1000ml of D_5W IV over 16h.

6. Administer all IV Mucomyst®/Acetadote® through a 0.22 micron filter.

TREATABLE BY HEMODIALYSIS OR HEMOPERFUSION

HD = hemodialysis; **HP** = hemoperfusion

Substance	Method of Choice	Indication
Ethylene glycol	HD	Altered mentation, hemodynamic instability, renal failure, metabolic acidosis, serum level >25mg/dl.
Isopropanol	HD	Hypotension, prolonged coma, level >400mg/dl.
Lithium	HD	Significant clinical symptoms, coma, seizures, myoclonus, severe tremor, renal failure, serum level >4mmol/liter (less if intoxication chronic).
Methanol	HD	Visual changes, altered mentation, metabolic acidosis, serum level >25mg/dl.
Salicylate	HD	Significant clinical symptoms: pulmonary edema, any neurologic sx, renal failure, worsening condition despite alkalinization, inability to alkalinize urine, metabolic acidosis, acute serum level approaching 100mg/dl, chronic serum level approaching 40-60mg/dl.
Theophylline	HP	Significant symptoms, seizures, acute serum levels approaching 80µg/ml or chronic levels approaching 40-60µg/ml.

PHONE RESOURCES FOR TOXICOLOGIC INFORMATION

Acute Poisoning

Your Regional Poison Control Center phone [   ]

If none available, Children's Hospital of Michigan Regional Poison Control Center, Detroit, MI

24 hours a day   *in Michigan* 800.222.1222
                                               outside Michigan 313.745.5711

Anthrax/Other Biowarfare Agents

USAMRIID   888.872.7443

Botulism

Local Health Dept
CDC   404.639.3311

Contaminated Food/Drugs

Food & Drug Administration, 5600 Fishers La., Rockville, MD 20857
Drugs: *8am-4:30pm Eastern M-F*   301.594.1012
Food: *24 hours a day*   301.443.1240

Drugs, Chemicals, and Radiation in Pregnancy

Motherisk, Division of Clinical Pharmacology, Hospital for Sick Children, 555 University Ave., Toronto, Ontario M5G1X8
9am-5pm Eastern M-F   416.813.6780
Other times   416.813.5900

Hazardous Chemical Reports

National Response Center, U.S. Coast Guard Headquarters, Attention: FOIA G-TPS-2, Room 2611, 2100 Second Street S.W., Washington, D.C. 20593
24 hours a day   800.424.8802

Hazardous Spill Containment

CHEMTREC, 2501 M Street N.W., Washington, D.C. 20037
24 hours a day   800.424.9300
ATSDR Emergency Response Hotline   404.639.0615

Pesticides

National Pesticide Network, Texas Tech University Health Sciences Center, Thompson Hall, Room S129, Lubbock, TX 79430
8am-6pm Central M-F   800.858.7378

(continued on following page)

PHONE RESOURCES FOR TOXICOLOGIC INFORMATION *(cont.)*

Chemicals, Identification of

Poison Control Center (see above) *or*
American Chemical Society, 1120 Vermont Ave. N.W., Washington, D.C.
    20005
8:30am-5pm Eastern M-F   800.227.5558

Radiation Accident

REAC/TS   423.576.3131
After hours   423.481.1000

Toxic Waste Disposal

Environmental Protection Agency, Public Information Center, 401 M
    Street S.W., Washington, D.C. 20460
9am-4:30pm Eastern M-F   202.260.2080
Environmental Response Hotline information   201.321.6660

CAUSES OF METABOLIC ACIDOSIS

Increased anion gap (Na-Chloride-CO_2 content ≥16 mEq/liter)

Diabetic ketoacidosis
Alcoholic or starvation ketoacidosis
Renal failure
    Intoxications
        Salicylate
        Methanol
        Ethylene glycol
        Paraldehyde
Lactic acidosis
    Inadequate oxygen delivery
        Shock (septic or hypovolemic)
        Generalized seizures
        Carbon monoxide poisoning
        Hypoxemia
    Failure to utilize oxygen
        Phenformin
        Diabetes mellitus
        Isoniazid overdose
        Iron overdose
    Unknown causes
        Hepatic cirrhosis
        Pancreatitis
        Pregnancy, especially with toxemia
        Chronic renal failure

Normal anion gap (Na-Chloride-CO_2 content <16mEq/liter)
    GI Loss of Bicarbonate
        Diarrhea
        Small bowel or pancreatic drainage or fistula
        Ureterosigmoidostomy
        Anion exchange resins
        Ingestion of $CaCl_2$ or $MgCl_2$

(continued on following page)

CAUSES OF METABOLIC ACIDOSIS *(cont.)*

Renal Loss of Bicarbonate
  Early renal failure
  Carbonic anhydrase inhibitors
  Renal tubular acidosis
  Hyperparathyroidism
  Hypoaldosteronism
Miscellaneous
  Dilutional acidosis
  Ingestion of NH_4 or HCl
  Sulfur ingestion

CAUSES OF METABOLIC ALKALOSIS

GI disorders
  Vomiting
  Gastric drainage
  Villous adenoma of the colon
  Chloride diarrhea
Diuretic
Correction of chronic hypercapnia
Cystic fibrosis
Hyperaldosteronism/Bartter's syndrome
Cushing's syndrome
Excessive licorice intake
Severe potassium depletion
Absorbable alkali administration
Milk-alkali syndrome
Massive plasma transfusion
Non-parathyroid hypercalcemia
Glucose ingestion after starvation
Large doses of carbenicillin or penicillin

CAUSES OF RESPIRATORY ALKALOSIS

Anxiety
Fever
Hypoxia
Chronic hepatic insufficiency
Hyperthyroidism
Sympathomimetics
Pulmonary embolus

CAUSES OF RESPIRATORY ACIDOSIS

CNS trauma or hemorrhage
Chest wall trauma
Pickwickian syndrome (severe obesity)
Chronic obstructive pulmonary disease
Neuropathic hypoventilation (e.g., ALS, myasthenia, polio)
Myopathies
Hypophosphatemia
Sedation: narcotics, barbiturates, benzodiazepines

CAUSES OF MIXED ACID-BASE DISTURBANCES

Metabolic Acidosis/Respiratory Acidosis

Cardiac arrest
Pulmonary edema

Metabolic Acidosis/Respiratory Alkalosis

Salicylate overdose
Sepsis

ACID-BASE NOMOGRAM

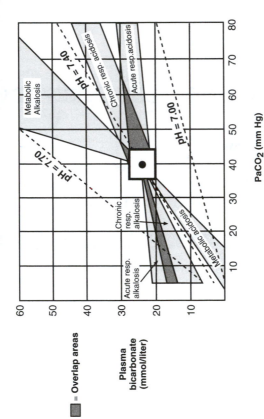

Figure 5-1 Acid-base nomogram, derived from the formulae beginning facing this page. Central square = area of normality for pCO_2, and bicarbonate ±4 units. A mixed acid-base disorder should always be considered, because on the nomogram it may mimic a single acute disorder. (Reproduced with permission from Schrier, ed., *Renal and Electrolyte Disorders*, 3rd edition, Little and Brown, 1986.)

Acid-Base Assessment Formulae

1. For **acute respiratory acidosis** or **alkalosis:**
   - *Is change in pH appropriate for acute change in $paCO_2$?*
   $\triangle$pH (from 7.40) = ($\triangle paCO_2$ − 40mm Hg) × .007

2. For **respiratory alkalosis:**
   - *Is bicarbonate concentration appropriate for change in $paCO_2$?*
   Acute:
   24 − bicarbonate = range of 1 to 3 × (40 − $paCO_2$/10)
       Bicarbonate should not fall below 18mmol/liter
   Chronic:
   24 − bicarbonate = range of 2 to 5 × (40 − $paCO_2$/10)
       Bicarbonate should not fall below 14mmol/liter

3. For **respiratory acidosis:**
   - *Is bicarbonate concentration appropriate for change in $paCO_2$?*
   Acute:
   Rise in bicarbonate = (40 − $paCO_2$/10). Appropriate range ±3.
   Chronic:
   Rise in HCO_3^- = (40 − $paCO_2$/10). Appropriate range ±4.

4. For checking the appropriateness of respiratory compensation in metabolic disorders:
   a. In **metabolic acidosis:**
      - *Is compensatory change in $paCO_2$ appropriate for degree of acidosis as expressed by drop in bicarbonate?*
      40 − $paCO_2$ = range of 1.0 to 1.5 × (24 − bicarbonate)
      Expect $paCO_2$ to be 26 to 36.5mm Hg
   b. In **metabolic alkalosis:**
      - *Is compensatory change in $paCO_2$ appropriate for degree of alkalosis as expressed by rise in bicarbonate?*
      40 − pCO_2 = range of 0.25 to 1.0 × (bicarbonate − 24)

5. For determining whether a mixed disorder is present:
   Delta gap = (Calculated anion gap − 12)/(24 − bicarbonate)
   Result ≥6 indicates:
   a. A mixed high anion gap metabolic acidosis plus a primary metabolic alkalosis; *or*
   b. A mixed high anion gap metabolic acidosis plus a chronic respiratory acidosis; *or*
   c. A non-acidotic high anion gap state (such as with excess penicillin administration).
   Result ≤−6 indicates:
   a. A mixed high anion gap metabolic acidosis plus a normal anion gap metabolic acidosis; *or*

(continued on following page)

ACID-BASE NOMOGRAM *(cont.)*

   b. A mixture of high anion gap metabolic acidosis plus chronic respiratory alkalosis plus hyperchloremia acidosis; *or*

   c. A high anion gap acidosis with a preexisting low anion gap state (such as hypoalbuminemia or para-proteinemia).

6. For venous blood gases:

   $PvCO_2$ normally 6-7mm Hg more than $paCO_2$;

   CO_2 content 2.5-3.0mm Hg more than arterial;

   Bicarbonate 1mmol/liter more than arterial.

ACUTE RENAL FAILURE VS. PRE-RENAL AZOTEMIA

Test	Azotemia	Renal Failure
Urine osmolality	>500	<400mOsm/kg
Urine sodium	<20	>40mEq/L
Urine creatinine/plasma creatinine	>40	<20
Renal failure index	<1	>2
Fractional excretion of sodium	<1	>2
Urine sediment	Normal or occ granular casts	Brown granular casts, cellular debris

$$\text{Creatinine clearance (ml/min)} = \frac{[(140 - \text{age}) \times \text{lean body weight in kg}]}{[\text{serum creatinine in mg/dl} \times 72]}$$

$$\text{Renal failure index} = \frac{U[Na]}{(U[Cr]/P[Cr])}$$

$$\text{Fractional excretion of sodium} = \frac{(U[Na]/P[Na])}{(U[Cr]/P[Cr]) \times 100}$$

U = urine   **P** = plasma   **Na** = sodium   **Cr** = creatinine

HEIGHT SURFACE AREA WEIGHT

Body Surface Area Nomogram

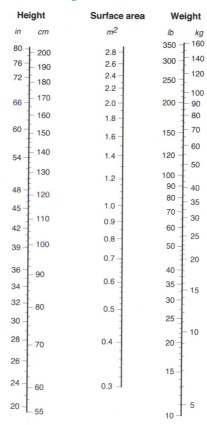

Figure 5-2 *To determine body surface area:* find height in centimeters or inches on left-hand scale and weight in pounds or kilograms on the right-hand scale. A straight line joining these points will cross the middle scale at the body surface area in meters squared.

DETROIT MEDICAL CENTER ALGORITHM FOR ASSESSING EXPOSURE TO BLOODBORNE VIRUS

(Unless noted otherwise, assumes donor HIV+ by hx or rapid testing—see pp. 123-124 for further details)

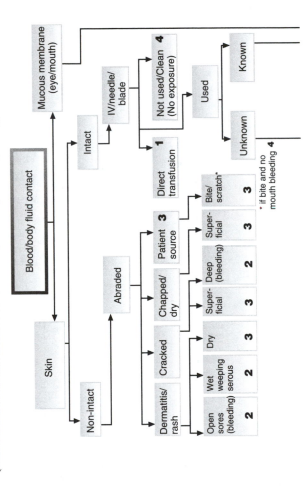

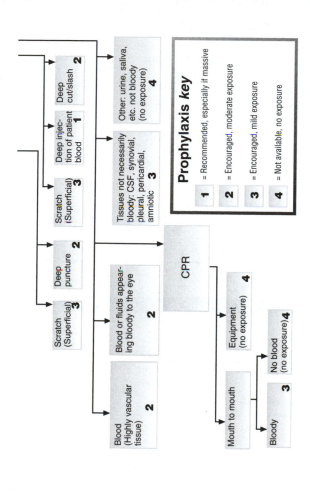

Figure 5-3 *Disclaimer:* this protocol was designed specifically for healthcare workers at the Detroit Medical Center (DMC). To those outside the DMC: the protocol should not be construed as recommending any specific course in cases of blood/body fluid exposure. Please consult responsible individuals/protocols at your institution. This protocol may at any time be modified or superseded by a new protocol.

Content within the figure:

Scratch (Superficial) **3**
Deep puncture **2**
Scratch (Superficial) **3**
Deep injection of patient blood **1**
Deep cut/slash **2**

Blood (Highly vascular tissue) **2**
Blood or fluids appearing bloody to the eye **2**
Tissues not necessarily bloody: CSF, synovial, pleural, pericardial, amniotic **3**
Other: urine, saliva, etc. not bloody (no exposure) **4**

CPR

Equipment (no exposure) **4**
Mouth to mouth
Bloody **3**
No blood (no exposure) **4**

Prophylaxis key

1 = Recommended, especially if massive exposure
2 = Encouraged, moderate exposure
3 = Encouraged, mild exposure
4 = Not available, no exposure

SYNOVIAL FLUID IN ACUTE ARTHRITIS

Diagnosis	Appearance	WBC/mm³	PMN %	Glucose*
Normal	Straw-colored, clear	<200	<25	~100
Degenerative joint disease	Slightly turbid	<2000	<25	~100
Traumatic arthritis	Straw-colored, bloody, or xantho-chromic	~2000	<25	~100
Rheumatoid arthritis	Turbid	5000-50,000	>65	~75
Other types of inflammatory arthritis	Turbid	5000-50,000	>50	~75
Acute gout or pseudogout	Turbid	5000-50,000	>75	~90
Septic arthritis	Very turbid or purulent	10,000-100,000	>80	<50
Tuberculous arthritis	Turbid	~25,000	Variable	<50

*% of blood level

CEREBROSPINAL FLUID IN MENINGITIS

Diagnosis	Glucose	Protein	WBC/mm³	PMN %	Pressure Opening (mm H_2O)
Normal	45-80	15-45	<5	0	<150
Bacterial	<40	>200	>1000	80	>300
Viral	>40	<200	<1000	<30	200
Fungal/TB	<40	>200	<500	<30	300

Values may vary with early meningitis or with atypical organisms.

HEMOPHILIA A AND B TREATMENT

The hemophilias cause joint, soft tissue, retroperitoneal, and central nervous system bleeding.

I. Basic Principles

Do: listen to patient: he/she knows his/her disorder best; contact patient's hemophilia treater; avoid unnecessary invasive procedures, IM injection, aspirin/other NSAIDs for pain relief; employ adequate pain control (po or IV opiates are often necessary for joint/soft tissue bleeds.)

Do not: refrain from necessary invasive diagnostic procedures; ensure adequate factor concentrate has been administered, then proceed.

II. Obtain an Accurate History Concerning:

A. Hemophilia type: Hemophilia A (Factor VIII deficiency) affects 80%, hemophilia B (Factor IX deficiency) 20% of patients (essential in determining appropriate factor concentrate).

B. Severity of disease:
1. *Severe (<1% factor activity):* frequent unprovoked bleeding, with spontaneous hemarthrosis, soft-tissue hemorrhage, CNS hemorrhage.
2. *Moderate (2%-5% factor activity):* occasional spontaneous, frequent trauma-induced bleeding in sites, similar to those with severe disease.
3. *Mild (>5% factor activity):* injury- or invasive procedure–induced bleeding.

III. Replace Coagulation Factor Always:

A. If patient has new headache, has altered mental status, or has sustained trauma or before any invasive diagnostic procedure.

B. Unless patient has already received adequate factor dose (many patients self-treat or receive home treatment).

IV. Select Appropriate Factor Concentrate.

Current care standards mandate use of safest recombinant factor products.

A. *Hemophilia A* (labs: prolonged PTT, low Factor VIII level)

Factor pharmacokinetics: $T^{1}/_{2} = 12h$.

Administer as: bolus IV loading dose followed by continuous infusion (preferable for severe injuries or surgical procedures); repeat bolus Q 8-12h.

Dose selection:
1. *Life-threatening bleeds* (CNS or retroperitoneal bleed, severe injury,

(continued on following page)

HEMOPHILIA A AND B TREATMENT *(cont.)*

surgical procedure): 45-50U/kg bolus, then 5-10U/kg/h by continuous
infusion or repeat bolus Q 8-12h.
2. *"Routine" bleeds* (hemarthrosis, hematuria, minor soft tissue):
   20-25U/kg bolus, repeat Q 8-12h as needed.

Factor concentrate choices:
1. *Recombinant products:* ReFacto®, KoGENate FS®, Helixate FS®,
   Recombinate®, Bioclate®, KoGENate®.
2. *Alternative therapy for mild/moderate hemophilia A:* Desmopressin
   nasal spray or solution (DDAVP, Stimate®): 1 spray/nostril or
   0.3μg/kg in 50ml 0.9% NaCl IV over 30min. Repeat Q 24h if necessary (use with great caution in pts >45y.o. or with cardiac histo-
   ries).
3. *Adjunctive therapy:* ε-aminocaproic acid (Amicar®): 1-4g po or IV Q
   4-6h (antifibrinolytic agent assists in preventing rebleeding).

**B. Hemophilia A with inhibitor antibody to Factor VIII and non-
hemophilic patients with acquired Factor VIII inhibitors**
Consult hematology immediately.

Factor concentrate choices:
1. *Replacement products* (useful when inhibitor titer<25 Bethesda U):
   High-dose Factor VIII: 100-400 U/kg bolus followed by repeat bolus
   Q 6-8h or 15-40U/h infusion; *or* Porcine Factor VIII (Hyate:C®):
   100-150U/kg Q 6-8h IV.
2. *"Bypass products"* (designed to bypass inhibitor target): rFactor
   VIIa (NovoSeven®): 75-90μg/kg Q 2-3h IV; *or* "Activated" prothrombin complex concentrates (Feiba-VH Immuno®): 50-75U/kg Q 6-8h
   (monitor PT and decrease dose or increase dosing interval if PT
   <5; use with caution in elderly patients).

C. Hemophilia B (labs: long PTT, low Factor IX level)
Factor pharmacokinetics: $T^1/_2$ = 18-24h.
Administer as: bolus followed by continuous infusion (preferred for
severe injury or surgical procedure); repeat bolus Q 15-18h.
Note: DDAVP is of no benefit in hemophilia B.

Dose selection:
1. *Life-threatening bleeds* (CNS or retroperitoneal bleed, severe injury,
   surgical procedure): 50-65U/kg bolus, then 7-12U/kg/h by continuous infusion or repeat bolus (25-30U/kg) Q 18-24h.
2. *"Routine" bleeds* (hemarthrosis, hematuria, minor soft tissue):
   25-30U/kg IV bolus, repeated Q 8-12h as needed.

Factor concentrate choices:
1. Recombinant Factor IX (BeneFix®).
2. *Adjunctive therapy:* ε-aminocaproic acid (Amicar®): 1-4g po or IV Q
   4-6h (antifibrinolytic agent assists in preventing rebleeding).

(continued on following page)

D. Hemophilia B with Factor IX inhibitor or anaphylactic allergy to Factor IX infusion

Consult hematology immediately.

Factor concentrate choices:

1. "Activated" prothrombin complex concentrates (Feiba-VH Immuno®): 50-75U/kg Q 6-8h (monitor PT and decrease dose or increase dosing interval if PT <5; use with caution in elderly). *These are absolutely contraindicated in patients with anaphylactic allergy to Factor IX; or*

2. rFactor VIIa (NovoSeven®): 75-90μg/kg Q 2-3h (sole choice for anaphylactic Factor IX allergy)

V. Remember: women with two affected genes can have hemophilia; severely affected male patients may have no family history; many adult hemophilia patients are HIV- and hepatitis C–infected.

VI. Refer patients to the nearest Comprehensive Hemophilia Treatment Center. Call Hemophilia Foundation of Michigan (800.482.3041) or National Hemophilia Foundation (800.424.2634) for listings. Detroit Medical Center Comprehensive Treatment Center: 313.745.9082 or call 313.745.0203, pager 1325.

VON WILLEBRAND DISEASE TREATMENT

VWD is a common autosomal bleeding disorder of men and women that causes bruising; epistaxis; and gingival, gastrointestinal, and uterine bleeding.

I. Obtain an accurate history: if no clear previous diagnosis, send labs: Factor VIII, vWF activity and antigen, platelet aggregation test. Type I: quantitative defect, mild; Type II: qualitative defect, variable; Type III: severe

II. Treatment:

Minor bleeding in mild Type I disease: desmopressin (DDAVP – dosing on p. 78) IV or nasal spray; *and/or* ε-aminocaproic acid 1-4g po/IV Q 4-6h.

Minor to major bleeding in Types I, II, III disease: vWF concentrate (Humate-P®), 25 (minor) to 100 (severe) U/kg IV, repeated Q 12-24h until bleeding controlled, *and* ε-aminocaproic acid, 1-4g po/IV Q 4-6h.

III. Refer patients to Comprehensive Hemophilia Treatment Center – see information above. Detroit Medical Center Hemophilia Treatment Center: 313.745.9082 or 313.745.0203, pager 1325.

MANAGEMENT OF THERAPEUTIC WARFARIN OVERDOSE

Clinical Situation	Guidelines
INR >therapeutic but <5.0, no clinically significant bleeding, rapid reversal not indicated	Lower the dose or omit the next dose; resume warfarin at the same or lower dose when INR is therapeutic. If the INR is only minimally above therapeutic range, dose reduction may not be necessary.
INR >5.0 but <9.0, no clinically significant bleeding	*Patients with no additional risk factors for bleeding:* omit next 1-2 doses warfarin, monitor INR more frequently, resume at lower dose when INR therapeutic. *Patients at increased risk of bleeding:* omit next warfarin dose, give vit. K1 1.0-2.5mg po. Patients requiring more rapid reversal before urgent surgery or dental extraction: vit. K1 2-4mg po. If INR still high at 24h, give vit. K1 1-2mg po.
INR >9.0, no clinically significant bleeding	*No clinically significant bleeding:* vit. K1 5-10mg po. Closely monitor INR. If not markedly reduced by 24-48h, may repeat vit. K1 dose. Resume at lower dose when INR therapeutic.
Serious bleeding at any elevation of INR	Vit. K_1 10mg slow IV *and either* FFP *or* recombinant factor Vlla. May repeat vit. K Q 12h prn.
Life-threatening bleeding	Vit. K_1 10mg slow IV *and either* prothrombin complex *or* recombinant factor Vlla. Repeat if necessary, depending on INR.

Adapted from: *Chest* 2004; 126(Suppl):213S.

WARFARIN INTERACTIONS

Drug classes in **bold type.** *If the drug you are interested in is not listed, do not assume lack of effect: look for further info.*

Drugs Causing Increased PT/INR

acetaminophen, alcohol, allopurinol, aminosalicylic acid, amiodarone, aspirin, azithromycin, **Beta-Blockers,** cefamandole, cefazolin, cefoperazone, cefotetan, cefoxitin, ceftriaxone, **Parenteral Cephalosporins,** chenodiol, chloramphenicol, chloral hydrate, chlorpropamide, cholestyramine, cimetidine, ciprofloxacin, clarithromycin, clofibrate, cyclophosphamide, danazol, dextran, dextrothyroxine, diazoxide, diclofenac, dicumarol, diflunisal, disulfiram, doxycycline, erythromycin, ethacrynic acid, fenoprofen, fluconazole, **Fluoroquinolones,** fluorouracil, fluoxetine, flutamide, fluvoxamine, glucagon, halothane, heparin, ibuprofen, ifosfamide, indomethacin, influenza virus vaccine, itraconazole, ketoprofen, ketorolac, levamisole, levothyroxine, liothyronine, lovastatin, **Macrolides,** mefenamic acid, methimazole, methyldopa, methylphenidate, methylsalicylate ointment (topical), metronidazole, miconazole, moricizine hydrochloride, nalidixic acid, **Narcotics,** naproxen, neomycin, **NSAIDS,** norfloxacin, ofloxacin, olsalazine, omeprazole, **Oral Diabetes Agents,** oxaprozin, oxymetholone, paroxetine, IV penicillin G, pentoxifylline, phenylbutazone, phenytoin, piperacillin, piroxicam, prednisone, propafenone, propoxyphene, propranolol, propylthiouracil, quinidine, quinine, ranitidine, sertraline, simvastatin, stanozolol, **Steroids,** streptokinase, sulfamethizole, sulfamethoxazole, sulfinpyrazone, sulfisoxazole, sulindac, tamoxifen, **Tetracyclines,** thyroid, ticarcillin, ticlopidine, tissue plasminogen activator (t-PA), tolbutamide, trimethoprim/sulfamethoxazole, urokinase, valproate, vitamin E, zafirlukast, zileuton

Drugs Causing Decreased PT/INR

6-mercaptopurine, alcohol, aminoglutethimide, amobarbital, **Antacids,** azathioprine, **Barbiturates,** butabarbital, butalbital, carbamazepine, chloral hydrate, chlordiazepoxide, chlorthalidone, cholestyramine, corticotropin, cortisone, cyclophosphamide, dicloxacillin, **Estrogen-Containing Steroids,** ethchlorvynol, glutethimide, griseofulvin, haloperidol, meprobamate, methimazole, moricizine hydrochloride, nafcillin, **Oral Contraceptives,** paraldehyde, pentobarbital, phenobarbital, phenytoin, prednisone, primidone, propylthiouracil, ranitidine, rifampin, secobarbital, spironolactone, sucralfate, trazodone, vitamin C (high dose), vitamin K

ISOLATION STRATEGIES AND CONTAGIOUS PERIODS FOR INFECTIOUS DISEASES

Disease	Precautions	Contagious Period
AIDS	Routine	Blood and body fluids should be considered infective with parenteral exposure
Campylobacter	* §	Until organisms can no longer be isolated from stool
Cholera	* §	Unknown
Clostridial myonecrosis	§	Until lesions are no longer draining
Diphtheria	SR M Go Gl	Until 2 cultures 24h apart from both nose and throat are negative
H. influenzae	SR M	Until 24h after initiation of effective antibiotic therapy
H. simplex		
Neonatal	SR M §	Duration of illness
Mucocutaneous	SR M §	For severe cases only – duration of illness
CNS	Routine	Special precautions unnecessary
Hepatitis A	* §	From 2wk before symptoms; minimum 1wk after onset of jaundice
Hepatitis B & C	Routine	HBsAg$^+$ state indicates infectivity for hepatitis B
Influenza	SR M §	Duration of illness
Measles	SR M	From 7d after exposure to 4d after onset of rash
Meningococcus	SR M	Until 24h after initiation of effective antibiotic therapy
Mumps	SR M	From 7d before parotid swelling to 9d after first symptoms
Pertussis	SR M	From first sx to 3wk later or 5d after start of erythromycin
Plague	SR M Go Gl	Until 72h after initiation of effective antibiotic therapy
Rabies	SR M Go Gl	Duration of illness
Rubella	SR M #	From 7d after exposure to 7d after onset of rash
Congenital	SR M #	Until 1 year of age unless nasopharyngeal and urine cultures are negative after 3 months of age

82

Condition	Precautions	Duration
Salmonellosis	*§	Until 3 stools after cessation of antibiotics are negative
Shigellosis	*§	Until 3 stools after cessation of antibiotics are negative
Staphylococcus		
Pneumonia	SR M §	Until 48h after start of effective antibiotic therapy
Skin	SR M §	Until open wounds have resolved
Strep skin (group A)	§	Until 24h after initiation of effective antibiotic therapy
Tuberculosis	SR M	From onset of sx until drug treatment reduces organisms found in sputum and cough is decreased
Varicella		
Chicken pox	SR M Go Gl	From 24h before rash until all lesions are crusted
Local zoster	§†	Until rash has resolved
Dissem. zoster	SR M Go Gl	Until rash has resolved
Yersiniosis	*§	Unknown

SR = single room   **M** = mask   **Go** = gown   **Gl** = gloves
Routine = universal precautions
*SR for patients with fecal incontinence or poor hygiene only
§Go, Gl only if contact with infective material likely
†Add SR, M if immunocompromised
#Add Go, Gl if immunocompromised

CHAPTER 6

PEDIATRIC REFERENCE

APGAR SCORING

Criterion	0	1	2
Heart rate	Absent	<100	>100
Respiratory	Absent	Slow or irregular	Good crying
Muscle tone	Limp	Some flexion of extremities	Active motion
Reflex irritability (catheter in nares)	No response	Grimace	Cough or sneeze
Color	Blue, pale	Extremities blue, body pink	Completely pink

Take at 1min and 5min after birth. **Results:** 8-10: normal infant; 4-7: mild to moderate impairment; 0-3: severely depressed.

TUBE AND LARYNGOSCOPE SIZES

Age	ET Tube*	Blade	Levine	Foley	Chest Tube Air	Chest Tube Fluid
	(IN MM)		(FRENCH)		(FRENCH)	
Neonatal	3.0	0	8	5–6	10–12	12
6 months	3.5–4.0	1	10	8–10	12	16–20
1 year	4.0–4.5	1	10	8–10	12–16	16–20
2 years	4.5–5.0	2	12	8–10	12–16	16–20
4 years	5.0–5.5	2	14	8–10	16–20	20–25
6 years	5.5–6.0	2	14	8–10	16–20	20–25
8 years	6.0–6.5	2–3	14	10–12	16–20	20–25
10 years	6.5–7.0	3	16	10–12	16–20	20–25
12 years	7.0–7.5	3	16	10–12	24–28	28–32
14 years	7.5–8.0	3	18	12–16	24–28	28–32

*Uncuffed tube unless >10 years old or tube size >6.0 mm

Pediatric Fever Algorithm 0-60 days Old
Temp greater than 38°C or 100.4°F

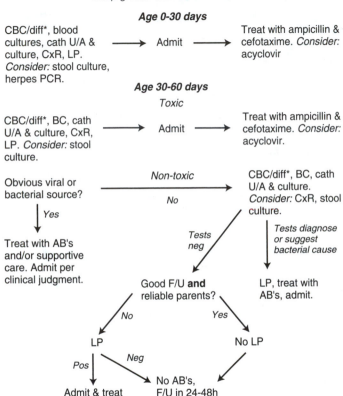

Notes for pediatric fever algorithms on this and facing page
* Positive CBC: WBC >15K or < 3.5 K, or absolute neutrophils <0.5K.
† High risk for UTI: urinary sx present, *or* hx UTI, *or* hx renal disease, *or* **boys** <6mo. old, *or* **boys** <1y.o. and uncircumcised, *or* **girls** <1y.o.

Figure 6-1   Pediatric fever algorithm, 0-60 days old.

Pediatric Fever Algorithm 2-36 Months Old
Temp greater than 38.5°C or 101.3°F

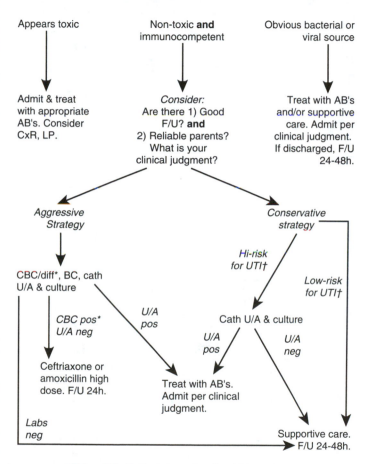

Figure 6-2 Pediatric fever algorithm, 2-36 months old.

HEMOGLOBIN AND MCV, BY AGE

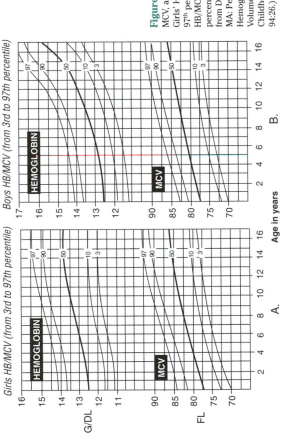

Figure 6-3 Hemoglobin, MCV, and WBC by age. A: Girls' HB/MCV (from 3rd to 97th percentiles). B: Boys' HB/MCV (from 3rd to 97th percentiles). (Reproduced from Dallman PR, Simes MA: Percentile Curves for Hemoglobin and Red Cell Volume in Infancy and Childhood. *J Pediatr* 1979; 94:26.)

WBC COUNT BY AGE

Age	WBC*
Term	9-30
2wk	5-20
1mo	5-19.5
2mo	5-19.5
6mo	6-17.5
6mo-2yr	6-17
2-6yr	5-15.5
6-12yr	4.5-13.5
12-18yr:	
Male	4.5-13.5
Female	4.5-13.5

*Per cu mm. Range = mean ± 2SD.

GIRLS' HEAD CIRCUMFERANCE

Girl's Head Circumference

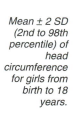

Mean ± 2 SD (2nd to 98th percentile) of head circumference for girls from birth to 18 years.

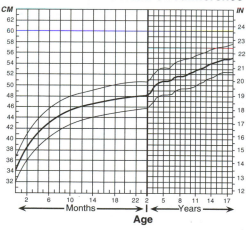

Figure 6-4   Girls' head circumference. Mean ± 2 SD (2nd to 98th percentile) of head circumference for girls from birth to 18 years. (From Nelhaus: *Pediatrics* 1968; 41:106.)

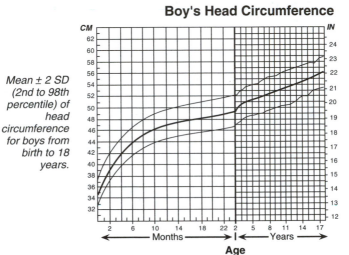

Figure 6-5 Boys' head circumference. Mean ± 2 SD (2nd to 98th percentile) of head circumference for boys from birth to 18 years. (From Nelhaus: *Pediatrics* 1968; 41:106.)

GIRLS' WEIGHT AND LENGTH, BIRTH TO 36 MONTHS

Girls Weight and Length Birth to 36 Months

From 5th to 95th percentile

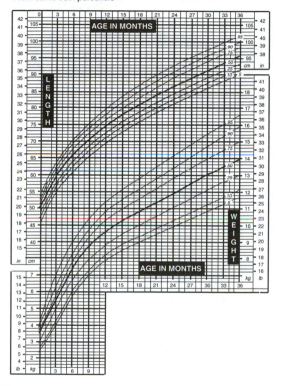

Figure 6-6 Girls' weight and length, birth to 36 months, from 5th to 95th percentiles. (Adapted from: Hamill PVV, Drizid TA, Johnson CL, Reed RB, Roche AF, Moore WM: Physical Growth: National Center for Health Statistic percentiles. *Am J Clin Nutr* 1979; 32:607-629. Data from the National Center for Health Statistics [NCHS], Hyattsville, MD.)

BOYS' WEIGHT AND LENGTH, BIRTH TO 36 MONTHS

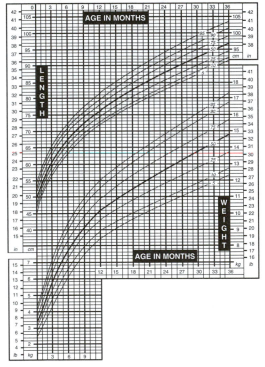

Boy's Weight and Length Birth to 36 Months

From 5th to 95th percentile

Figure 6-7   Boys' weight and length, birth to 36 months, from 5th to 95th percentiles. (Adapted from: Hamill PVV, Drizid TA, Johnson CL, Reed RB, Roche AF, Moore WM: Physical Growth: National Center for Health Statistic percentiles. *Am J Clin Nutr* 1979; 32:607-629. Data from the National Center for Health Statistics [NCHS], Hyattsville, MD.)

CHAPTER 7

TREATMENT OF SPECIFIC DISEASES

TREATMENT OF SPECIFIC DISEASES

Disease	Regimen
Abortion, threatened	Check CBC, blood type. If Rh negative, give *RhoGam* 300µg IM.
Adrenal insufficiency	*If diagnosis unconfirmed:* Dexamethasone 4mg IV *and* fludrocortisone 0.1mg po. *If known dx:* Hydrocortisone 200mg IV. *In all cases:* Replace sodium/water deficits, treat hypoglycemia with D50 IV **preferred** *or* glucagon 1-2mg IM.
Alcohol withdrawal	[(Diazepam 5-10mg IV Q 10min *or* lorazepam 1-2mg Q 10min *or* phenobarbital 260mg IV, then 130mg Q 30min) *and* thiamine 100mg *and* magnesium 4g IV over 30min-1h]. *Therapeutic goal is light sedation/autonomic stability. Severe cases (~25%) may require massive doses (diazepam >200mg/ lorazepam >20mg).*
Allergic reaction	*Mild* *Child/adult:* Diphenhydramine 1mg/kg po/IM/IV *and* (cimetidine 3mg/kg po/IV *or* ranitidine 1 mg/kg po/IV). *Moderate* *Child/adult: As for simple, but add* methylprednisolone 2mg/kg IV *or* prednisone 1mg/kg po. If discharged, continue oral Rx for 48-72h. *Anaphylaxis or anaphylactoid reaction* *Child/adult:* [(Epinephrine 1:1000 sltn 0.01ml/kg SC/IM, max 0.5ml {0.5mg}); *or for severe cases* (epinephrine 1:1000 sltn 1ml {0.1mg} slow IV); *then if still refractory* (epinephrine 1:10,000 sltn 0.1ml/kg IV, max 3ml {0.3mg}) *and* (methylprednisolone 2mg/kg IV) *and* (diphenhydramine

(continued on following page)

TREATMENT OF SPECIFIC DISEASES *(continued)*

Disease	Regimen
Allergic reaction *(cont'd)*	1mg/kg IV) and (cimetidine 3mg/kg IV *or* ranitidine 1mg/kg IV)]. *If laryngeal edema:* Racemic epinephrine 2.25% sltn 0.5ml nebulized. *If bronchospasm:* Albuterol *and* ipratropium nebulized. *If hypotension:* NS bolus/infusion. *If refractory hypotension:* Albumin 5% sltn IV *and/or* (dopamine *or* norepinephrine infusion).
Amebiasis	*Asymptomatic* *Child/adult:* Paromomycin 8-12mg/kg (max 500mg) po TID for 7d. *Diarrhea/dysentery* *Child/adult:* Metronidazole 12-17mg/kg (max 500-750mg) po TID for 7d, then paromomycin 8-12mg/kg (max 500mg) po TID for 7d. *Extra-intestinal (e.g., hepatic abscess)* *Child/adult:* Metronidazole 12-17mg/kg (max 750mg) po/IV for 10d, then paromomycin 8-12mg/kg (max 500mg) po TID for 7d. *Start metronidazole IV, then switch to po.*
Anaphylactic shock	*Child/adult:* [Epinephrine 1:1000 0.01ml/kg up to 0.5ml (0.5mg) IM while starting IV; then, if still in shock, epinephrine 1:10,000 0.1ml (0.01mg)/kg up to 3ml (0.3mg) IV over several min] *and* diphenhydramine 1mg/kg IV *and* [ranitidine 1mg/kg IV *or* cimetidine 3mg/kg IV] *and* methylprednisolone 2mg/kg IV. *For laryngeal edema:* Racemic epinephrine 0.5ml in 3cc NS aerosolized. *For wheezing:* Albuterol aerosol *and/or* aminophylline loading. *For hypotension:* Dopamine *or* norepinephrine. *Use adrenergics with care in elderly or those with heart disease or HTN.*
Aortic dissection	*Adult:* [(Nitroprusside: start 0.3µg/kg/min, titrate to max 5.0µg/kg/min) *and* (esmolol 500µg IV bolus, then 50-200µg/kg/min *or* metoprolol 5mg IV Q 2min for 3 doses, then 2-5mg/h IV infusion);

(continued on following page)

Disease	Regimen
	or [labetalol 20mg IV, then 40-80mg IV Q 10min, until desired effect, max 300mg, then maintain at 1-2mg/h]. *If β-blocker contraindicated:* Trimethaphan 1-2min mg/min IV. *Therapeutic goals:* HR 60-80, SBP 100-120.
Arthritis, septic	Arthrocentesis is required for all suspected cases. Initial antibiotic(s) guided by likely age-related organisms/G-stain. Use vancomycin in place of PCNs if high prevalence of MRSA or if PCN allergy.
<3mo.	(Nafcillin *or* oxacillin) and (3rd-gen ceph *or* tobramycin, *or* amikacin *or* gentamicin). **Etiol:** *Staph. aureus*, group B *Strep.*, Enterobacteriaceae.
3mo.-14y.o.	(Nafcillin *or* oxacillin *or* vancomycin) *and* (3rd-gen ceph). **Etiol:** *Staph. aureus*, group A *Strep.*, *S. pneumoniae*, *H. influenzae*.
Gonococcal	Ceftriaxone 1gIM/IV QD; *or* cefotaxime 1g IV Q 8h; *or* ceftizoxime 1g IV Q 8h.
14y.o.-adult (not gonococcal)	(Nafcillin *or* oxacillin) *and* (3rd-gen ceph *or* ciprofloxacin). **Etiol:** *N. gonorrhoeae, Staph. aureus, Streptococcus* spp., Enterobacteriaceae.
Prosthetic joint, post-op, post-arthrocentesis, or post-IVDU	Vancomycin *and* (ciprofloxacin *or* aztreonam *or* cefepime *or* piperacillin *or* piperacillin/tazobactam *or* ticarcillin *or* ticarcillin/clavulanate). **Etiol:** *Staph. epidermidis, Staph. aureus*, Enterobacteriaceae, *P. aeruginosa.*
Atrial fibrillation	Follow the usual indications for emergency cardioversion. Control ventricular response as necessary with diltiazem, digoxin, or β-blocker. For all heparin/Coumadin candidates, ascertain whether contraindications exist. If they do, start on ASA—all pts with afib should receive antithrombotic Rx. Recent data questions the superiority of attempt to convert/maintain sinus rhythm over rate control (NEJM 347; 1834).

TREATMENT OF SPECIFIC DISEASES (continued)

Disease	Regimen
New onset (within 48h)	Typical hx: new-onset palpitations or acute CHF with rapid rate. Start heparin or LMWH *and* Coumadin 5mg po QD, aiming for INR 2-3. Cardioversion may be attempted within 48h.
Of unknown/ uncertain duration	Start heparin *or* LMWH *and* Coumadin 5mg po QD. If cardioversion strategy elected and TEE negative for thrombosis, cardiovert within 48h. If thrombosis present, continue heparin and DC when INR 2-3. Bring patient back in 1mo. for elective cardioversion.
Chronic management of anticoagulation	*High risk for embolic CVA defined by any one of:* age >75y.o.; hx of prior TIA or stroke; uncontrolled HTN (SBP >160); CHF in past 3mo.; depressed LV function; prosthetic heart valve. For patients on Coumadin, aim for INR 2-3. *Adult <65y.o., no high risk:* Aspirin 325mg po QD. *Adult <65y.o., high risk:* Coumadin. *Adult 65-75y.o., no high risk:* Aspirin 325mg po QD or Coumadin. *Adult 65-75y.o., high risk:* Coumadin. *Adult >75y.o., low/high risk:* Coumadin.
Bell's palsy	*Adult:* (Prednisone 1mg/kg po QD for 5d, then taper to 5mg po BID over 5d) *and* (for 10d acyclovir 400mg po TID *or* valacyclovir 1g po BID *or* famciclovir 250mg po TID). Brain CT unnecessary if presentation is typical. Most common cause is herpes simplex; in endemic areas, consider Lyme disease. Ophthalmic lubricant/tape for eye closure at night reduces risk of corneal abrasions.
Bites	*Principles:* (1) Consider x-ray for fx/FB, (2) tetanus prophylaxis (see p. 46), (3) consider rabies prophylaxis (see p. 133), (4) admit for grossly infected wounds, esp. hand or if extensive tissue destruction, (5) if no active infection, treat with ABs for 5d.
Bat, raccoon, skunk	Low risk of infection, antibiotic prophylaxis rarely indicated. *If treatment elected:* Amoxicillin/ clavulanate *or* doxycycline. **Etiol:** Unclear.

See index for generic names of proprietary meds

Disease	Regimen
Cat	Amoxicillin/clavulanate; *or* cefuroxime; *or* doxycycline.
	Etiol: *Pasteurella multocida, Staph. aureus, Streptococcus.*
Dog	Amoxicillin/clavulanate; *or* [clindamycin *and* (fluoroquinolone or TMP-SMX)].
	Etiol: *P. multocida, S. aureus, Streptococcus, Bacteroides, Fusobacterium, Peptostreptococcus,* Enterobacteriaceae, *Capnocytophaga canimorsus.*
Human	Amoxicillin/clavulanate **preferred for prophylaxis;** *or* ampicillin/sulbactam; *or* cefoxitin; *or* ticarcillin/clavulanate; *or* piperacillin tazobactam; *or* [clindamycin *and* (ciprofloxacin *or* TMP-SMX)].
	Etiol: Polymicrobial, often with *E. corrodens, S. aureus,* Viridans strep, *Corynebacterium, Bacteroides, Peptostreptococcus.*
Monkey	Amoxicillin/clavulanate; *or* cefuroxime; *or* [clindamycin and (fluoroquinolone or TMP-SMX). **If suspicion of Herpesvirus simiae:** *Adult:* (*For 14d* valacyclovir 1g po BID or acyclovir 800mg po 5 times/d).
	Etiol: *E. corrodens, P. multocida, S. aureus, Streptococcus.*
Pig (swine)	Amoxicillin/clavulanate; *or* 3rd-gen ceph.; *or* ticarcillin/clavulanate; *or* ampicillin/sulbactam; *or* imipenem.
	Etiol: *Pasturella, Bacteroides, Streptococcus, Proteus.*
Rat	Amoxicillin/clavulanate; *or* doxycycline.
	Etiol: *Spirillum minus, bacillus moniliformis.*
Bullous pemphigoid	*Adult:* [Prednisone 40-60mg po QD *and* (azathioprine 1mg/kg po QD *or* cyclophosphamide 1mg/kg po QD)]. *Consult dermatology.*
Bursitis, septic	Amoxicillin/clavulanate; *or* dicloxacillin; *or* cloxacillin; *or* oxacillin; *or* nafcillin; *or* methicillin; *or* 1st-gen ceph; *or* vancomycin; *or* [ciprofloxacin *only if* ≥18y.o. *and* rifampin].
	Etiol: *Staph. aureus.*

See index for generic names of proprietary meds

TREATMENT OF SPECIFIC DISEASES *(continued)*

Disease	Regimen
Candida	
Oral (thrush) – **no HIV**	*Child <3y.o.:* Nystatin suspension (100,000U/ml) 1cc po QID for 7d after lesions disappear. *Child 3y.o.-adult:* Clotrimazole troches; *or* nystatin susp; *or* (adult *only*) fluconazole 100mg po single dose.
Oral (thrush) or **esophageal –** **with HIV**	*Child:* Clotrimazole troches; *or* nystatin susp; *or* (3-13y.o. only) fluconazole 10mg/kg (max 200mg) po, then 24h later start 3-6mg/kg po QD. *Child 13y.o.-adult:* Clotrimazole troches; *or* nystatin susp; or fluconazole 200mg po, then 24h later start 100mg po QD (up to 400mg/d has been used); *or* ketoconazole 200-400mg po QD; *or* itrachonazole solution 100mg (10ml) swish and swallow BID. *Treat AIDS patients for at least 3wk and for at least 2wk after resolution of symptoms.*
Skin	Topical clotrimazole; *or* miconazole; *or* nystatin.
Vaginitis	See *"vaginitis."*
Cellulitis/ **erysipelas**	*Outpatient* *Child/adult:* 1st-gen ceph; *or* dicloxacillin; *or* azithromycin; *or* clarithromycin; *or* clindamycin; *or* ciprofloxacin only if ≥18y.o. or levofloxacin only if ≥18y.o. *Inpatient* *Child/adult:* 1st-gen ceph; or nafcillin; *or* oxacillin; *or* ciprofloxacin only if ≥18y.o.; *or* (levofloxacin only if ≥18y.o. and clindamycin); *or* ampicillin/sulbactam. *Severe or recurrent disease:* Piperacillin/tazobactam; *or* ticarcillin/clavulanate; *or* imipenem; *or* meropenem. *Diabetes* *Outpatient and/or mild disease:* Ampicillin/sulbactam; *or* 2nd-gen ceph; *or* 3rd-gen ceph. *Severe disease/inpatient:* Imipenem; *or* meropenem; *or* ertapenem.

Disease	Regimen
Cerebral edema	*Child/adult:* Elevate head of bed to 30°. Intubation with mild hyperventilation (pCO2 28-32) may be beneficial. ***If signs of herniation:*** *Child/adult:* Mannitol 0.5-1g/kg IV, then 0.25-0.5g/kg IV Q 2-3h prn. ***If due to neoplasm:*** *Child/adult:* Dexamethasone 0.15mg/kg IV, then 0.1mg/kg IV Q 6h.
Cerebrovascular accident	
General	(R/O hypoglycemia—may mimic CVA) and (perform stat CT scan) *and* (if symptoms ≤3h, activate stroke team or obtain stat neuro consult) *and* (use NIHSS to determine severity of deficit—see pp. 31-33) *and* (treat seizures with benzodiazepines *and* phenytoin) *and* (avoid overhydration or administration of dextrose-containing sltns).
HTN management	Goal is 10-20% max reduction, treat *only* if SBP >220, DBP >120 or MAP >130mmHg with (labetalol 10-20mg IV, then 20-40mg IV Q 20min prn, max total 150mg); *or* (enalapril 0.625-2.5mg IV Q 20min, max total 5mg).
Refractory HTN	Nitroprusside 0.5-10μg/kg/min, titrate to desired effect. If thrombolytic candidate, goal is SBP <185 and DBP <110mm Hg. If BP does not respond to labetalol 10-20mg IV Q 20min for max 2 doses and nitroglycerin paste 1-2, do not thrombolyse.
Transient ischemic attack	Aspirin 325mg po QD *or* aspirin/dipyridamole *or* clopidogrel. Full anticoagulation with only heparin indicated for atrial fibrillation or if cardiac mural thrombus present.

TREATMENT OF SPECIFIC DISEASES (continued)

Disease	Regimen
Ischemic stroke	Evaluate for eligibility for thrombolysis—risk of intracranial hemorrhage ~6.5%. If contraindicated, treat as for TIA. Criteria for thrombolysis (must meet all): (1) time of onset <3h, (2) no hemorrhage on CT, (3) age >18y.o. Thrombolysis excluded for any of: (1) sustained BP >185/110, (2) minor or improving symptoms, (3) platelet count <100K, (4) Hct <25, (5) glucose <50 or >400, (6) prolonged PT or PTT, (7) heparin given past 48h, (8) witnessed seizure at stroke onset, (9) ischemic CVA past 90d, (10) closed-head injury past 90d, (11) any prior hx of hemorrhagic CVA, (12) major surgery past 14d; (13) GI bleed past 21d, (14) recent MI, (15) LP past 7d, (16) suspicion of aortic/carotid dissection. *If thrombolysis indicated:* Alteplase total dose 0.9mg/kg (max 90mg), give 10% as IV bolus, then 90% IV over 1h. Intra-arterial administration during angiography is an alternative. Hold anticoagulation for ≥24h after thrombolysis. Monitor BP Q 15min for 2h after infusion, then Q 30min for 6h, then Q 1h for 16h. If SBP >180mm Hg or DBP >105 mmHg, start labetalol as previously or if refractory nitroprusside as previously.
Hemorrhagic stroke	Supportive care, control increased ICP. Treat BP elevations as above. Consider seizure prophylaxis with phenytoin IV load/maintenance. Consult neurosurgeon—hematoma evacuation may be indicated, esp. cerebellar. Altered mental status common. Strongly associated with antecedent HTN. Fatal in ~50% of cases.
Subarachnoid hemorrhage	Consult neurosurgeon stat. Give supportive care, prevent cerebral vasospasm with nimodipine 60mg po or per NG Q 4h.

See index for generic names of proprietary meds

Disease	Regimen
Chancroid	*Adult:* Azithromycin 1g po single dose **preferred;** *or* ceftriaxone 250mg IM single dose **preferred;** *or* erythromycin 500mg po QID for 7d **preferred;** *or* ciprofloxacin 500mg po BID for 3d.
***Chlamydia trachomatis* urethritis/ cervicitis**	*General:* Evaluate for concurrent STDs and empirically treat for GC. *Child <45 kg:* Erythromycin base 12.5mg/kg po QID for 14d; *or child >45kg:* Azithromycin 1g po single dose; *or only if >8y.o:* Doxycycline 100mg po BID for 7d. *Adult:* Azithromycin 1g po single dose **preferred;** *or (for 7d* doxycycline 100mg po BID *or* ofloxacin 300mg po BID *or* levofloxacin 500mg po QD *or* erythromycin base 500mg po QID *or* erythromycin ethylsuccinate 800mg po QID). *Pregnant: (For 7d* erythromycin base 500mg po QID **preferred;** *or* amoxicillin 500mg po TID **preferred;** *or* erythromycin ethylsuccinate 800mg po QID); *or* (erythromycin base 500mg po for 14d).
Cholecystitis/ Cholangitis	*Child/adult:* Ampicillin/sulbactam; *or* piperacillin/ tazobactam; *or* ticarcillin/clavulanate; *or* ertapenem; *or* meropenem; *or* imipenem; *or* [(metronidazole) *and* (3rd-gen ceph *or* aztreonam *or* ciprofloxacin *only if* ≥18y.o.)]. Optimize volume status, administer antiemetics as needed, provide appropriate pain control.
Coronary syndromes, acute	*Unstable angina or continuing ischemia* ASA 325mg po *and* (NTG 0.4mg SL Q 5min prn, up to 3 doses; if pain continues, start IV at 20µg/min, may increase by 5-10µg/min Q 5min prn—**warning:** NTG may cause hypotension, esp. if RV ischemia/infarction present) *and* (O2 2L NC if saturation <95%) *and* (metoprolol 5mg IV Q 5min for 3 doses prn, followed in 15min by 25-50mg po Q 12h; *other β-blockers also effective, target HR 60-70, avoid if 2° or 3° heart block, PR interval >22msec, active bronchospasm, SBP <100 or recent cocaine use) and* (enoxaparin 1mg/kg

(continued on following page)

See index for generic names of proprietary meds

TREATMENT OF SPECIFIC DISEASES *(continued)*

Disease	Regimen
Coronary syndromes, acute *(cont'd)*	SC [may precede with 30mg IV] *or* (heparin 60U/kg IV, then 12U/kg/h IV) *and* (morphine 2-4mg IV Q 15min prn for persistent pain). *If moderate-severe HTN:* Captopril 6.5mg po once *or* enalaprilat 1.25-2.5mg IV Q 15min, max total 5mg.

Non-ST segment elevation MI (NSTEMI)

As for unstable angina and after consulting cardiology, consider clopidogrel 300mg po once *and consider* (tirofiban 0.4µg/kg/min IV over 30min, then 0.1µg/kg/min IV); *or* (eptifibatide 180µg/kg IV, then 2 µg/kg/min IV).

ST segment elevation MI (STEMI)

As for unstable angina and in consultation with cardiology, arrange for reperfusion within 60min of arrival with [cardiac catheterization **preferred if available**] *or* [*thrombolyse with* (alteplase 15mg IV bolus, then infusion of 0.75mg/kg, max 50mg, over 30min, then 0.5mg/kg, max 35mg, over 60min) *or* (reteplase 10U IV bolus, then 10U in 30min) *or* (tenecteplase weight-based dosing: for <60kg, 30mg; for 60-70kg, 35mg; for 70-80kg, 40mg; for 80-90kg, 45mg; for >90kg, 50mg IV) *or* (anistreplase 30mg IV over 2-5min) *or* (streptokinase 1.5 million U over 60min)]. **If cath lab:** Clopidogrel 300mg po *and* (tirofiban dosing as for NSTEMI *or* eptifibatide dosing as for NSTEMI). **If thrombolytics:** (1) continue heparin/LMWH during thrombolysis; (2) concurrent use of GP IIb/IIIa inhibitors controversial.

Thrombolytic contraindications: *Absolute:* Active internal bleeding, ischemic CVA within 1yr, any hx of hemorrhagic CVA, intracranial neoplasm, suspected aortic dissection, known hypersensitivity to any thrombolytic. *Previous use of streptokinase precludes use of this agent. Relative:* BP ≥180/110, trauma or closed-head injury within 2-4wk, concurrent Coumadin/warfarin with INR >2, known bleeding diathesis, recent internal bleeding, major surgery within wk, active PUD, pregnancy, noncompressible venous or arterial puncture, prolonged CPR.

Disease	Regimen
Croup (laryngotra-cheobron-chitis)	*Child:* IV hydration prn *and* humidified O$_2$ mist *and* (nebulized racemic epinephrine 0.5ml of 2.25% *or* epinephrine 0.5cc of 1:1000 sltn Q 20min, repeat prn) *and* (dexamethasone 0.6mg/kg, max 10mg, po/IM/IV) *and/or* (budesonide 2mg nebulized once). *Consider admission if stridor, dyspnea, tachycardia, hypoxia, or cyanosis persists; for marked distress at home or in ED; or if F/U not assured.*
Diabetes mellitus	*Uncomplicated hyperglycemia, new-onset* *Child:* Admit to assess treatment response and for education. Regular insulin/hydration as clinical state dictates. *Adult:* Check renal function/ electrolytes *and* hydrate with NS *and* administer regular insulin as needed to reduce glucose to <300. If stable for DC, start glyburide *or* glipizide 5-10mg po QD *or* if sulfa allergy or obese, metformin 500mg po BID. If pt was symptomatic from DM, clinic f/u indicated in 1-2d. *Diabetic ketoacidosis (DKA)* *Child:* (NS 20ml/kg IV over 1h, reassess and repeat Q 1h as needed for signs of dehydration but do not exceed 40ml/kg in 1st 4h) *and* (regular insulin 0.1U/kg/h). Monitor MS for signs of cerebral edema. *Adult:* (NS 1L IV bolus, further hydration as indicated) *and* (regular insulin 0.1U/kg IV bolus *is optional,* then 0.1U/kg/h IV) *and* (add KCl 20-40mEq/L to IV if K <5.5 and adequate renal function). When glucose <250, change IV to D5 0.45% NS. Bicarbonate indicated only if pH ≤7.0. Determine and treat precipitating conditions. *Hyperglycemia, hyperosmolar, nonketotic* *Adult:* Hydrate with (*if signs of dehydration, oliguria, or Na <150:* 0.9 NS 2-3 L over 1-2h IV *or if Na >150 and no oliguria or signs of dehydration:* 0.45 NS 2-3 L over 1-2h IV) *and* (regular insulin 0.05-0.1U/kg IV bolus *is optional,* then 0.05-0.1U/kg/h IV) *and* (add KCl as for DKA). After NS bolus, change IV to 0.45% NS. When glucose <250, change IV to D5/0.45% NS and maintain glucose at 200-300 to prevent cerebral edema. Dx/treat precipitating factors.

TREATMENT OF SPECIFIC DISEASES *(continued)*

Disease	Regimen
Diverticulitis	**PO/IV:** [Metronidazole *and* (TMP/SMX *or* 1st-gen ceph *or* 2nd-gen ceph *or* ciprofloxacin)]. **IV:** [Cefoxitin *and* (gentamicin *or* tobramycin *or* amikacin)]; *or* [(metronidazole *or* clindamycin) *and* (amikacin *or* gentamicin *or* tobramycin)]; *or* [ticarcillin/clavulanate *with or without* (amikacin *or* gentamicin *or* tobramycin)]; *or* [impenem *with or without* (amikacin *or* gentamicin *or* tobramycin)]. **Etiol:** *Enterobacteriaceae, Bacteroides, Enterococci.*
Duodenal ulcer relapse (*Eradication of Helicobacter pylori*)	*Adult:* [(Omeprazole 20mg po BID *or* lansoprazole 30mg po BID) *and* amoxicillin 1g po BID *and* clarithromycin 500mg po BID for 7d]; *or* [tetracycline 500mg po QID *and* Pepto Bismol 2 tabs (302mg) po QID *and* metronidazole 500mg po TID *and* omeprazole 20mg po BID for 7d].
Dysfunctional uterine bleeding	Medroxyprogesterone acetate (*Provera*) 10-20mg po for 7-10d; *or* norethindrone (*Micronor*) 10mg po for 7d. Bleeding stops in 2-4d. If more rapid onset desired, a combo OCP such as mestranol 50μg/ norethindrone 1mg (*Ortho-Novum 1/50* or *Norinyl 1+50*) or ethinyl estradiol 50μg/norgestrel 0.5mg (*Ovral*) 4 tablets po QD for 5-7d. Bleeding controlled within 12-24h. *Check preg test. Do not use OCPs if obese, age >35, or smoker.* Advise patients to expect 6-7d of heavy bleeding with cramping 3-7d (for progesterones) or 2-4d (for OCPs) after treatment stops.
Dystonic reaction, acute	*Child:* Diphenhydramine 1.25mg/kg IM/IV, then 1.25 mg/kg po QID for 3d; *or* benztropine 0.02-0.05mg/kg IM/IV *only if* >3y.o., then 0.02-0.05mg/kg po BID for 3d. *Adult:* Diphenhydramine 50mg IM/IV, then 50mg po QID for 3d; *or* benztropine mesylate (*Cogentin*) 1mg IM/IV, then 1-2mg po BID for 3d.

Disease	Regimen
Eclampsia	MgSO$_4$ 4-6g IV over 1h, then 2g/h IV. Monitor for loss of reflexes/resp. depression. *If DBP >110 after MgSO$_4$:* Hydralazine 5mg IV, then 5-10mg IV Q 20min prn; *or* labetalol 20mg IV, then 20-40mg IV Q 10min prn. *If seizures do not respond to MgSO$_4$:* Diazepam 5-10mg IV; *or* lorazepam 1-2mg IV.
Endocarditis	Obtain 3 sets blood cultures with at least 1h between 1st and last before starting ABs. *Native valve* *Child:* Vancomycin and gentamicin. *Adult:* (PCN G 20MU/d continuous infusion or div. Q 4h IV *or* ampicillin 12g/d continuous infusion or div. Q 4h IV) *and* (gentamicin 1mg/kg IV Q 8h). *IVDU* *Adult:* Vancomycin 15mg/kg (max 2g) Q 12h and (gentamicin 1mg/kg IV Q 8h). *Prosthetic valve* *Child:* Vancomycin and gentamicin. Rifampin as for adults below. *Adult:* (Vancomycin 15mg/kg [max 2g] IV Q 12h) *and* (gentamicin 1mg/kg IV Q 8h). May add rifampin 600mg po QD but this is generally withheld pending susceptibility testing. *Urgent surgical consultation indicated.*

Prophylaxis: *Conditions susceptible to endocarditis:* **High risk:** Any prosthetic valve; hx of endocarditis; surg. constructed systemic pulm. shunts or conduits; complex cyanotic congenital heart disease (e.g., single-ventricle states, transposition of the great arteries, tetralogy of Fallot). **Moderate risk:** Most other congenital cardiac malformations; acquired valve dysfunction (e.g., rheumatic heart disease); hypertrophic cardiomyopathy; mitral valve prolapse with valve regurg. or thickened leaflets. *Conditions for which prophylaxis is NOT indicated:* Isolated secundum atrial septal defect; hx of surgical repair of ASD, VSD, or patent ductus arteriosus (without residua beyond 6mo. old); history of CABG; mitral valve prolapse w/o regurg.; physiologic heart murmurs; history of Kawasaki's or of rheumatic fever without valve dysfunction; implanted cardiac pacer or defibrillator.

See index for generic names of proprietary meds

TREATMENT OF SPECIFIC DISEASES *(continued)*

Disease	Regimen

*Procedures with risk: **Dental:*** Extractions; periodontal procedures, including surgery, scaling and root planing, probing, and recall maintenance; dental implant placement and reimplantation of avulsed teeth; endodontic instrumentation or surgery only beyond the apex; subgingival placement of antibiotic fibers or strips; initial placement of orthodontic bands but not brackets; intraligamentary local anesthetic injections; prophylactic cleaning of teeth/implants where bleeding is anticipated. ***Other:*** Tonsillectomy and/or adenoidectomy; surgery that involves resp. mucosa; bronchoscopy with a rigid bronch; sclerotherapy for esoph. varices; esoph. stricture dilation; endoscopic retrograde cholangiography with biliary obstruction; biliary tract surgery; surgery that involves intestinal mucosa; prostatic surgery; cystoscopy; urethral dilation.

Antibiotics/dosing: *Give all initial po doses 1h prior and finish all initial IM/IV doses within 30min of procedure. **Dental, oral, upper resp. tract, or esoph. procedures:** Adult:* Amoxicillin 2g po. *Child:* Amoxicillin 50mg/kg po. <u>Unable to take po:</u> *Adult:* Ampicillin 2g IM/IV. *Child:* Ampicillin 50mg/kg IM/IV. <u>PCN/amoxicillin allergic</u>: *Adult:* Clindamycin 600mg po; *or* cephalexin 2g po; *or* cefadroxil 2g po; *or* azithromycin 500mg po; *or* clarithromycin 500mg po. *Child:* Clindamycin 20mg/kg po; *or* cephalexin 50mg/kg po; *or* cefadroxil 50mg/kg po; *or* azithromycin 15mg/kg po; *or* clarithromycin 15 mg/kg po. <u>Unable to take oral meds and PCN allergic</u>: *Adult:* Clindamycin 600mg IV; *or* cefazolin 500mg IV. *Child:* Clindamycin 20mg/kg IV; *or* cefazolin 25mg/kg IM/IV.

Genitourinary or gastrointestinal procedures: <u>High-risk conditions</u>: *Adult:* [Ampicillin 2g IV/IM *and* gentamicin 1.5mg/kg (max 120mg), then 6h later either ampicillin 1g IM/IV *or* amoxicillin 1g po]. *Child:* [Ampicillin 50mg/kg IM/IV *and* gentamicin 1.5mg/kg, then 6h later either ampicillin 25mg/kg IM/IV *or* amoxicillin 25mg/kg orally]. *If PCN/amoxicillin allergic*: *Adult:* [Vancomycin 1g IV *and* gentamicin 1.5mg/kg (max 120mg) IM/IV]. *Child:* [Vancomycin 20mg/kg IV over 1-2h *and* gentamicin 1.5mg/kg IV/IM]. <u>Moderate-risk conditions</u>: *Adult:* Amoxicillin 2g po; *or* ampicillin 2g IM/IV. *Child:* Amoxicillin 50mg/kg po; *or* ampicillin 50mg/kg IM/IV.

Disease	Regimen
Epididymitis	
GC or chlamydia (STD)	*Adult:* Ceftriaxone 250mg IM, then (*for 10d* doxycycline 100mg po BID *or* ofloxacin 400mg *or* levofloxacin 500mg po QD).
Age >35 or likely enteric organisms or allergic to cephalosporins and/or tetracycline	*Adult:* Ciprofloxacin 500mg po BID for 14d; *or* ofloxacin 400mg po BID for 10d; *or* levofloxacin 500mg po QD for 10d; *or* TMP-SMX 1 DS po BID for 14d. *Severe disease* *Adult:* Ampicillin/sulbactam; *or* piperacillin/tazobactam; *or* ticarcillin/clavulanate; *or* 3rd-gen ceph.
Epiglottitis	*Child/adult:* (Cefuroxime *or* cefotaxime *or* ceftriaxone *or* ampicillin/sulbactam) *and* (dexamethasone 0.15-0.3mg/kg IV QID). Nebulized racemic epinephrine 0.5ml of 2.25% sltn *and* dexamethasone 0.15-0.3mg/kg may reduce airway edema. *Secure airway early in children. If culture positive for H. influenzae, treat pt and household contacts with rifampin (see p. 258) to eliminate nasopharyngeal carriage.* **Etiol:** *Child: Staph. aureus, H. influenzae. Adult:* Group A *Strep., Staph. aureus, H. influenzae.*
Fasciitis, necrotizing	*Adult:* [(Clindamycin 600-900mg IV Q 6h) *and* (PCN G 4MU IV Q 4h *or* ampicillin 2g IV Q 4h *or* cefazolin 1-2g IV Q 8h)]; *or* [(2nd-gen ceph) *and* (ciprofloxacin 400mg IV Q 12h *or* levofloxacin 500mg IV QD *or* gatifloxacin 400mg IV QD *or* moxifloxacin 400mg IV QD)]; *or* [(vancomycin 1g IV Q 6h) *and* (metronidazole 500mg IV Q 6h) *and* (ciprofloxacin *or* levofloxacin *or* gatifloxacin *or* moxifloxacin)]. *Hallmark: pain out of proportion to skin findings. Extensive tissue destruction >common w perineal involvement (Fournier's gangrene). Aggressive hemodynamic resuscitation indicated; operative care is definitive.*

TREATMENT OF SPECIFIC DISEASES *(continued)*

Disease	Regimen
Gastroenteritis	*Most cases are self-limited and/or have viral etiology (Norwalk, rotavirus); care is supportive.* *Time of sx related to pathogen inoculation:* 1-6h: Staphylococcal enterotoxin, *B. cereus* type I, enterotoxigenic *E. coli* 8-24h: *C. perfringens, B. cereus* type II, *enteroinvasive E. coli, Salmonella, V. parahaemolyticus* 24-72h: *Shigella, V. cholera*, enteroinvasive and enterohemorrhagic *E. coli, Plesiomonas shigelloides* 2-7d: *Yersinia* sp., *C. jejuni, Aeromonas hydrophila* *Protracted sx or immunocompromised:* *Cryptosporidium, Cyclospora cayetanensis, Isospora belli, Giardia lamblia*
Severe case (≥6 BMs/d, temp ≥101°, tenesmus, bloody stool)	*Child:* (*For 5-7d* cefixime 4mg/kg po BID *or* TMP/SMX as trimeth. 4mg/kg po BID. *Adult:* (*For 3d* ciprofloxacin 500mg po BID *or* levofloxacin 500mg po QD *or* TMP/SMX 1 DS tab po BID). *If bloody stool but no fever, consider etiology E.coli O157: H7—ABs may increase chance of hemolytic uremic syndrome.* **Etiol:** *Salmonella, shigella, C. jejuni, E. coli* O157: H7, *E. histolytica*
C. difficile **toxin** (*suspect if severe sx and recent antibiotics*)	*Child:* Metronidazole 7-12 mg/kg (max 500mg) po TID; *or* vancomycin 10 mg/kg po (max 125mg) Q 6h. *Adult:* Metronidazole 500mg po TID; *or* vancomycin 125mg po QID. *Treat for 10d. Send stool for toxin assay.*
Traveler's diarrhea	*Adult:* Azithromycin 1g po once; *or* levofloxacin 500mg po once; *or* ciprofloxacin 500mg po BID for 3d. *ABs may shorten course, most are self-limited.* **Etiol:** *Tox. E. coli, Campylobacter jejuni, salmonella, shigella, C. difficile, amebiasis.*

Disease	Regimen
Giardiasis	*Child/adult:* Metronidazole 5mg/kg (max 250mg) po TID for 5d; *or* furazolidone 1.5mg/kg (max 100mg) po QID for 10d *(only Rx available in liquid form)*; *or* tinidazole 50mg/kg for one dose (max 2g); *or* quinacrine 2mg/kg (max 100mg) po TID after meals for 5d; *or* albendazole 400mg po QD for 5d.
Glaucoma, acute angle closure	*Mild-moderate:* Timolol 0.5% 1 drop Q 30min *and* apraclonidine 1% 1 drop Q 30min for 2 doses *and* pilocarpine 2-4% 1 drop Q 15min. *Severe cases:* As for mild-moderate *and* [acetazolamide 250-500mg IV *and* (chilled glycerol 50% sltn 1ml/kg po *or* mannitol 1-2 g/kg IV over 45min.] *Manage pain aggressively. Emergent ophthalmologic consult for all cases.*
Gonorrhea	Evaluate for concurrent STDs, treat empirically for *Chlamydia*. Avoid fluoroquinolones if infection acquired where resistance is common: Asia, Pacific Islands, Hawaii, or California.
Uncomplicated urethral, cervicitis, or anorectal infection	*Child <45kg:* Ceftriaxone 125mg IM single dose; *or* spectinomycin 40mg/kg (max 2g) IM single dose. *Child ≥45kg-adult:* Ceftriaxone 125mg IM single dose **preferred**; *or* cefixime 400mg po single dose **preferred**; *or* ciprofloxacin 500mg po single dose **preferred**; *or* levofloxacin 250mg po single dose **preferred**; *or* ofloxacin 400mg po single dose **preferred**; *or* spectinomycin 40mg/kg (max 2g) IM single dose; *or* ceftizoxime 500mg IM single dose; *or* cefotaxime 500mg IM single dose; *or* norfloxacin 800mg po single dose; *or* lomefloxacin 400mg po single dose; *or* gatifloxacin 400mg po single dose. *Pregnant patient:* Ceftriaxone 125mg IM single dose; *or* cefixime 400mg po single dose; *or* spectinomycin 40mg/kg (max 2g) IM single dose).

TREATMENT OF SPECIFIC DISEASES *(continued)*

Disease	Regimen
Conjunctivitis	Ceftriaxone 1g IM single dose *and* copious irrigation with NS.
Disseminated	*Child:* Ceftriaxone 50mg/kg (max 1g) IV QD. *Adult:* Ceftriaxone 1g IM/IV QD **preferred**; *or* cefotaxime 1g IV Q 8h; *or* ceftizoxime 1g IV Q 8h; *or* ciprofloxacin 400mg IV Q12h; *or* ofloxacin 400mg IV Q 12h; *or* levofloxacin 250mg IV QD; *or* spectinomycin 2g IM Q 12h. *Treat IV for 24-48h, then for 7d:* cefixime 400mg po BID *or* ciprofloxacin 500mg po BID *or* ofloxacin 400mg po BID *or* levofloxacin 500mg po QD.
Meningitis/ endocarditis	*Adult:* Ceftriaxone 1-2g IV Q 12h.
Ophthalmia neonatorum	Ceftriaxone 25-50mg/kg (max 125mg) IM/IV single dose. Consider admission; DC only after consultation.
Pharyngitis	Ceftriaxone 125mg IM single dose; *or* ciprofloxacin 500mg po single dose.
Gout, acute attack	*Adult:* [Indomethacin 50-75mg po, then 50mg po Q 6h until 24h after relief, then 50mg po Q 8h for 3 doses, then 25mg po Q 8h for 3 doses]; *or* colchicine 1.2mg po, then 0.5-0.6mg po Q 2h until relief or GI sx (max 6mg). *Optional:* Triamcinolone 5-10mg intra-articular for small joints or 20-40mg IA for large joints may be beneficial.
Granuloma inguinale	*Adult:* Doxycycline 100mg po BID *or* TMP-SMX DS 1 tab po BID. *Treat for 3wk or until all lesions have healed. Rare in U.S.*
Headache *Cluster*	*Child/adult:* [100% oxygen by mask *and* 4% lidocaine instilled into affected side nares]; *or* migraine treatment (see below); *or* narcotics (see below).

See index for generic names of proprietary meds

Disease	Regimen
Migraine	*Adult:* Dihydroergotamine mesylate nasal spray (0.5mg/spray) 1 spray each nostril, repeat in 15min; *or* sumatriptan 6mg SC, may repeat in 1h; *or* sumitriptan nasal spray (10mg/spray) 1 spray each nostril; *or* sumitriptan 25mg po; *or* naratriptan 2.5mg po; *or* rizatriptan 10mg SL/po; *or* zolmitriptan 2.5mg po; *or* prochlorperazine 5-10mg IV/PR/po; *or* [metoclopramide 5mg IV with or without dihydroergotamine]. Refractory migraines may respond to dexamethasone 4-6mg IM/IV Q 6h. *For treatment failures, use narcotics (see below).*
Post LP (Spinal)	*Prevention:* Use small-gauge, blunt-tip needle; limit fluid removed; avoid lifting, bending, and squatting for 3d.
	Treatment: IV hydration; caffeine 500mg IVPB over 2h; narcotics (see below); epidural blood patch.
"Salvage" headache regimen	Morphine sulfate 0.1mg/kg IV/IM/SC Q 2h prn pain or hydromorphone 1mg SC/IM Q 2h prn. In patients habituated to opiates, larger doses may be needed.
Heart failure, acute	*With HTN:* [(Nitroglycerin 0.4mg SL for 3 doses; if not considerably improved, start IV infusion at 0.5-1μg/kg/min, titrate Q 1-2min, max 400 μg/min *and* furosemide 40-80mg IVP *or* double pt's oral dose/d up to 160mg). If no response to nitroglycerin, consider sodium nitroprusside 0.5-10μg/kg/min]; *or* [nesiritide 2μg/kg IV, then 0.01μg/kg/min, titrate up to 0.03μg/kg/min, continue infusion for 24h]; *or* [enalapril 0.625-2.5mg IV or captopril 25mg po/SL]. *With hypotension:* [Dobutamine 2-20μg/kg/min IV *with or without* dopamine 2-20μg/kg/min IV] *or* [milrinone 50μg/kg IV, then 0.375-0.75μg/kg/min].

TREATMENT OF SPECIFIC DISEASES *(continued)*

Disease	Regimen
Hemophilia	See p. 77.
Hepatitis, viral	Treatment generally supportive; hospital admission rarely required for acute episodes. Vaccinate susceptible populations/exposed persons to minimize disease transmission. Post-exposure prophylaxis is based on suspected viral subtype and extent of risk involved.
Hepatitis A (HAV)	*Incubation period:* 15-45d, mean 30d. *Post-exposure prophylaxis indicated:* Close personal contacts; day care center employees or attendees where a case of hep A has been dx'ed; or those with food consumption from a known source facility or restaurant. *Prophylax with: Child/adult:* Within 14d immune globulin (IG) 0.02ml/kg IM single dose. *No hep A specific globulin available.* *Pre-exposure prophylaxis indicated: 1st dose at least 15-30d before exposure for:* Travelers to developing countries, household and sexual contacts of persons infected with hep A, child day care employees, patients with chronic liver disease, illicit drug users, men having sex with men, institutional workers, hospital employees who may be exposed to hep A. *Prophylax with: Child 2-17y.o.:* HAV vaccine 0.5ml IM. *Adult:* HAV vaccine 1ml IM. *For all give 2nd dose in 6-12mo. Doses refer to either* Havrix *or* Vaqta.
Hepatitis B (HBV)	Incubation period: 30-180d, mean 60-90d. ***Post-exposure prophylaxis indicated:*** Health care workers with bodily fluid exposures involving percutaneous penetration or mucosal surface contact, or persons with unprotected sexual contact with confirmed source.

Disease	Regimen
	Prophylax with: Child/adult: Within 14d hepatitis B immune globulin (HBIG) 0.06ml/kg IM *and* hepatitis B vaccine (see p. 204 for dosing). *After completion of vaccination, assess antibody response with anti-HbsAg testing. If inadequate (≤10mIU/ml):* HBIG 0.06ml/kg IM *and* (re-initiation of vaccination series *or* HBIG second dose in 1 mo.).
	Pre-exposure prophylaxis with vaccine indicated: Dentists and oral surgeons; physicians and surgeons; nurses; paramedical personnel and custodial staff who may be exposed to the virus via blood or other patient specimens; dental hygienists and dental nurses; laboratory personnel handling blood, blood products, and other patient specimens; dental, medical, and nursing students; staff in hemodialysis units and hematology/oncology units; pts requiring frequent and/or large-volume blood transfusions or clotting factor concentrates; clients (residents) and staff of institutions for the mentally handicapped; classroom contacts of deinstitutionalized mentally handicapped persons who have persistent hepatitis B surface antigenemia and who show aggressive behavior; household and other intimate contacts of persons with persistent hepatitis B surface antigenemia; infants born to HBsAg-positive mothers whether HBeAg positive or negative.
Hepatitis C (HCV)	*Incubation period: 15-160d, mean 50d.* No currently accepted prophylactic regimens exists. Chronic cases may be treated with interferon and ribavirin.
Hepatitis D (HDV)	*Incubation period: 30-180d, mean 60-90d.* Requires concurrent HBV infection; thus prevention is HBV vaccination.
Hepatitis E (HEV)	*Incubation period: 14-60d, mean 40d.* Self-limited, mild sx. No vaccine available, no indication for IG.

TREATMENT OF SPECIFIC DISEASES *(continued)*

Disease	Regimen
Herpes simplex	

Herpes simplex

Bell's palsy — See p. 96 (Bell's palsy entry)

Encephalitis — *Child/adult:* Acyclovir 10mg/kg IV Q 8h for 14-21d.

Genital, primary — *Child >12y.o.-adult:* Acyclovir 400mg po TID; *or* valacyclovir 1g po BID; *or* famciclovir 250mg po TID. *Treat for 10d.* **Severe disease and/or immunocompromised:** Acyclovir 5mg/kg IV Q 8h.

Genital, recurrent — *Child >12y.o.-adult:* Acyclovir 400mg po TID for 5d or 800mg po TID for 2d; *or* valacyclovir 500mg po BID for 3-5d; *or* famciclovir 125mg po TID for 5d.

Genital, chronic suppression — *Child >12y.o.-adult:* Acyclovir 400mg po BID; *or* valacyclovir 500mg po BID; *or* famciclovir 125mg po BID. *Indicated if >10 episodes/yr or in pregnancy wk 36-40 only.*

Genital, immuno-compromised — *Use regimen for gingivostomatitis, immunocompromised.*

Gingivostomatitis — *Child <12y.o.:* Acyclovir 20mg/kg po QID for 7d. *Child >12y.o.-adult:* Valacyclovir 2g po Q 12h for 2d; *or* acyclovir 400mg Q 4h (5x/d) for 5d; *or* famciclovir 500mg po BID for 7d; *or* penciclovir 1% cream Q 2h while awake for 4d; *or* acyclovir 5% cream Q 3h (6x/d) while awake for 7d. ***Immunocompromised:*** Acyclovir 5-10mg/kg IV Q 8h for 7d; *or* acyclovir 400mg po TID for 14-21d.

Keratoconjunctivitis — *Child/adult:* Trifluridine 1% 1 drop Q 2h while awake, max 9 drops/d; *or* vidarabine 3% ophthalmic ointment apply 0.5 inch to lower conjunctival sac 5x/d while awake. *Treat for 14-21d.*

Disease	Regimen
Whitlow, herpetic	*Child >12y.o.-adult:* Treatment usually symptomatic, with dry dressing coverage to prevent spread of infection. ***If immunocompromised or recurrent:*** Acyclovir 400mg po TID for 10-14d.
Hypertension	Need for acute treatment based on sx and/or end-organ damage: cardiac ischemia, LV dysfunction, aortic dissection, renal failure, encephalopathy, CVA, retinal hemorrhage—not on BP alone.
New-onset, asymptomatic	Recheck after 30min of rest. If persistent and unrelated to pain/anxiety evaluate or arrange for evaluation for end-organ damage w/urinalysis, BUN/Cr, ECG if >50y.o., CxR. Acute BP lowering not indicated. Consider starting *for most patients* hydrochlorothiazide 12.5-25mg po QD; *or if CAD hx,* β-blocker; *or if DM or CHF hx,* ACE inhibitor; or *if CVA hx or >65y.o.,* Ca++ channel blocker.
Chronic, asymptomatic	Rebound HTN common if noncompliant, esp. with clonidine. *If noncompliant,* start baseline medications. *If compliant,* consider increased dose or addition of different class agent.
Symptomatic, non-specific mild (diastolic <115 mm Hg)	*Evaluate for end-organ damage. Acute management usually not required. When needed, consider* (labetalol 20mg IV, then 40-80mg IV Q 10min prn, max 300mg); *or* (hydralazine 5-10mg IV Q 20min prn); *or* (enalapril 0.625-2.5mg IV Q 20min, max 5mg); *or* (clonidine 0.1-0.2mg po Q 1h).
Cocaine-related	*Avoid β-blockers.* (Diazepam 5-10mg *or* lorazepam 1-2mg IV Q 5-15min) *and if necessary,* phentolamine 2.5-5mg IV Q 5min prn. **For refractory cases:** Nitroprusside 0.5-10μg/kg/min *or* nitroglycerin start at 5μg, titrate either as needed.

TREATMENT OF SPECIFIC DISEASES *(continued)*

Disease	Regimen
Hypertensive emergency (severe/acute end organ injury)	*Therapeutic goal: 20-30% reduction in MAP.* (Nitroprusside 0.5μg/kg/min, titrated to max 10mg/kg/min); *or* (labetalol 20mg IV, then 40-80mg IV Q 10min prn up to 300mg max); *or* (labetalol 20mg IV bolus then 2 mg/min IV, titrate prn); *or* fenoldopam 0.03-0.1μg/kg/min IV, titrate by 0.05-0.1μg/kg/min Q 15min to max of 1.6μg/kg/min IV; *or* nitroglycerin start at 5μg, titrate to max 200μg/min.; *or* nicardipine 2mg/h IV, titrate Q 15min, max 15mg/h; *or* esmolol 500μg/kg IV, then 50-200μg/kg/min IV.
Hyperthermia, malignant	*Child/adult:* Stop instigating medication, hyperventilate with 100% O2. Give dantrolene 1 mg/kg IV Q 5-10min (max 10 mg/kg total dose), until pt improves. Benzodiazepines for skeletal muscle relaxation reduce thermogenesis and rhabdomyolysis. *Prepare to treat hyperthermia, hyperkalemia, metabolic acidosis, DIC, myoglobinuria, and rhabdo. Avoid Ca++ channel blockers. Use procainamide for cardiac dysrhythmia as needed.* For management assistance, call the Malignant Hyperthermia Association of the United States: 1.800.644.9737.
Hyperthyroidism *(Thyroid storm)*	*Child:* (Propranolol 0.01-0.1mg/kg, max 1mg if <1y.o., max 3mg IV if >1y.o., *or if less severe disease,* propranolol 0.125-0.25mg/kg po Q 6h, target HR < 100) *and* (propylthiouracil [PTU] 2mg/kg po Q8h), *and 1h after PTU* (potassium iodide 50-250mg po TID). *Adult:* (Propranolol 1mg IV Q 5-10min, max 10mg to target HR < 100) *and* (PTU 800-1200mg po, then 300mg po Q 6h] *and* (dexamethasone 2mg IV Q 6h *or* hydrocortisone 100mg IV Q 8h) *and 1h after 1st PTU* (sodium iodide continuous infusion at 125mg/h *or* potassium iodide 5 drops po Q 6h *or* Lugol's iodine sltn 10 drops po Q 8h). *For all, supportive therapy incl. fluids, electrolyte repletion, and treatment of hyperpyrexia with acetaminophen, not aspirin, is essential.*

See index for generic names of proprietary meds

Disease	Regimen
Hypoglycemia	*Child <1y.o.:* D10 1-2ml/kg IV, then at 2ml/kg/h IV). *Child >1y.o.:* D25 2-4ml/kg IV, then D10 2-4ml/kg/h IV). *Adult:* D50 1-3 amps IV, repeat prn). **If no immediate IV access:** *Child:* Glucagon 0.025-0.1 IMmg/kg. *Adult:* Glucagon 1-2mg IM. **Related to sulfonylureas:** *Adult:* Octreotide 50-75μg IM/IV Q 6h. **For mild cases:** Oral glucose sltn/juice. *Admit when secondary to long-acting insulin* (Lantus) *or long-acting sulfonylurea.*
Hypothyroid myxedema coma	*Adult:* Send TSH and T4 levels, then (levothyroxine 500μg IV, then 25μg po/IV Q 6h) *and* (hydrocortisone 300mg IV, then 100mg IV Q 8h). *Supportive treatment essential. Avoid aggressive rewarming.*
Impetigo	*Child/adult:* Mupirocin 2% ointment to affected area TID *and* (erythromycin 7.5mg/kg, max 250mg, po QID *or* cephalexin 7.5-10mg/kg, max 500mg, po QID). *Treat for 7-10d.* **Bullous variant:** *Child/adult:* Dicloxacillin 10-12mg/kg, max 500mg, po QID. Mupirocin ointment as above optional. *Treat for 7-10d.*
Lice	
Body	Rx of pt usually not necessary. Discard clothing; if not possible, Rx clothing with 1% malathion *or* 10% DDT powder, or remove from body contact for 72h (until lice die). *Organism lives on clothing; leaves only for blood meals.*
Head or pubic (crabs)	Permethrin 5% or 1% liquid lotion, apply for 10min; *or* lindane 1% shampoo, apply for 4min, then wash off thoroughly (*do not use if preg. or < 2y.o.*); *or* pyrethrins with piperonyl butoxide (RID), apply and wash off in 10min. *After Rx, decontaminate clothing/bedding with washing machine hot cycle or with dry cleaning or by removing from bodily contact for 72h. Rx household and close and sexual contacts. Nit removal with nit comb or enzymatic remover is an important adjunct.*

See index for generic names of proprietary meds

TREATMENT OF SPECIFIC DISEASES *(continued)*

Disease	Regimen

Lyme disease

Tick bite
Do not use antibiotics for most bites. To be effective, risk of transmission needs to be ≥1%. Because transmission occurs in 10% of bites by infected ticks, ≥10% of local ticks need to be infected for antibiotics to be effective.

Early (erythema chronicum migrans, isolated facial palsy, 1st-degree heart block)
Child: Amoxicillin 17 mg/kg (max 500mg) po TID for 21d **preferred;** *or if ≥9y.o.:* Doxycycline 1-2mg/kg (max 100mg) po BID for 21d; *or* cefuroxime axetil 15mg/kg (max 500mg) po BID for 21d.
Adult: Doxycycline 100mg po BID for 21d **preferred;** *or* amoxicillin 500mg po TID for 21d; *or* cefuroxime axetil 500mg po BID for 21d.

Arthritis
Child: Amoxicillin 17mg/kg (max 500mg) po TID for 28d; *or if ≥9y.o.:* doxycycline 1-2mg/kg (max 100mg) po BID for 28d; *or* ceftriaxone 50-75mg/kg (max 2g) IV QD for 14-28d; *or* PCN G 300,000U/kg/d (max 18-24 million U) for 14-28d.
Adult: Doxycycline 100mg po BID for 28d; *or* amoxicillin 500mg po TID for 28d; *or* ceftriaxone 2g IV QD for 14-28d; *or* PCN G 18-24 million U/d IV for 14-28d.

Cardiac disease except 1st-degree heart block
Child: Ceftriaxone 50-75mg/kg (max 2g) IV QD for 14-21d; *or* PCN G 300,000U/kg (max 18-24 million U) IV/d for 14-21d.
Adult: Ceftriaxone 2g IV QD for 14-21d; *or* PCN G 18-24 million U IV/d for 14-21d.

Neurologic symptoms except isolated facial palsy
Child: Ceftriaxone 75-100mg/kg (max 2g) IV QD for 14-28d; *or* cefotaxime 50-67mg/kg IV Q 8h for 14-28d; *or* PCN G 300,000U/kg (max 18-24 million U) IV/d for 14-28d.
Adult: Ceftriaxone 2g IV QD for 14-28d; *or* cefotaxime 2g IV Q 8h for 14-28d; *or* PCN G 20-24 million U/d IV for 21d.

Disease	Regimen
Lymphogranuloma venereum	*Adult:* Doxycycline 100mg po BID for 21d **preferred**; *or* erythromycin base 500mg po QID for 21d; or sulfamethoxazole 500mg po QID for 21d.
Malaria *Treatment (~1000 U.S. cases/yr)*	Dx via blood smear. Treat all *P. vivax* and *P. ovale* with primaquine to prevent relapse. **Initial treatment of all species, chloroquine resistance assumed:** *Child:* [For 7d (quinine 8.5mg/kg po TID) *and* (doxycycline 1mg/kg, max 100mg, po BID *or* clindamycin 10mg/kg, max 900mg, po TID **preferred**)]; *or* [mefloquine 15mg/kg po, max 750mg, then 10mg/kg, max 500mg, po in 12h]; *or* [halofantrine† 8mg/kg, max 500mg, po Q 6h for 3 doses, repeat regimen in 1wk]; *or* [(artesunate† 4mg/kg/d po QD for 3d) *and* (mefloquine 15mg/kg po, max 750mg, then in 12h 10mg/kg, max 500mg, po)]. *Adult:* [For 7d (quinine 650mg po TID) *and* (doxycycline 100 po BID)]; *or* [For 7d (quinine 650mg po TID *and* clindamycin 900mg po TID) **preferred if preg.**] *or* [mefloquine 750mg po once, then in 12h 500mg po]; *or* [halofantrine† 500mg po Q 6h for 3 doses, repeat regimen in 1wk]; *or* [(artesunate† 4mg/kg/d po QD for 3d) *and* (mefloquine 750mg, then 500mg po in 12h)]. ***Chloroquine-sensitive P. falciparum, vivax, or ovale:*** *Child:* Chloroquine 10 mg/kg (max 600mg), then 5mg/kg (max 300mg) po in 6h, 24h, 48h; then primaquine as below. *Adult:* Chloroquine 1g po, then 0.5g po in 6h, 24h, 48h, then primaquine as below. ***All who are treated for P. vivax/ovale:*** *Child:* Primaquine 0.5mg (0.3mg base)/kg po QD for 14d. *Adult:* Primaquine 26.3mg (15mg base) po QD. *Treatment for 14d prevents relapse. Contraindicated if G6PD.*

(continued on following page)

See index for generic names of proprietary meds

TREATMENT OF SPECIFIC DISEASES *(continued)*

Disease	Regimen
Treatment (~1000 U.S. cases/yr) (cont'd)	***Severely ill/cannot tolerate po meds:*** *Child/adult:* [Quinidine gluconate 10mg/kg IV over 1-2h, then 0.02mg/kg/min IV]; *or* [quinidine dihydrochloride 20mg/kg IV over 4h, then 10mg/kg IV Q 8h, infuse in 2-4h]; *or* [artemether 3.2mg/kg IM, then 1.6mg/kg IM QD for 5-7d]. *Exchange transfusion may be indicated. Change to oral meds when improved.* †=*not available in United States.*

Prophylaxis   *In addition to drug regimens, protection should include:* Screens, nets, DEET 30-35%, permethrin spray on clothing/nets.

Areas with chloroquine sens. malaria (Central America west of the Panama Canal, the Caribbean, Mexico, parts of the Middle East and China): *Child:* Chloroquine 5mg/kg, max 500mg, po Q wk. *Adult:* Chloroquine 500mg po Q wk. *Start 1wk before arrival, continue for 4wk after leaving.*

Areas with chloroquine resistance (All other regions): *Child:* [Mefloquine: *<15kg,* 5mg/kg po; *15-19 kg,* 1/4 tab po; *20-30 kg,* 1/2 tab po; *31-45kg,* 3/4 tab po; *>45 kg,* 1 tab po. *Take Q wk, start 3wk before arrival, continue 4wk after leaving*]; *or* [atovaquone/proguanil (Malarone): *11-20kg,:* 62.5/25mg po; *21-30kg,* 125/50mg po; *31-40kg,* 187.5/75mg po; *>40kg,* 250/100mg (1 adult tab) po. *Take QD, start 1d before arrival, continue 1wk after leaving*]; *or* [doxycycline 2mg/kg, max 100mg, po QD. *Start 2d before arrival, continue 4wk after leaving*]. *Adult:* [Atovaquone 250mg/proguanil 100mg (Malarone) 1 tab po QD, *start 1d before arrival, continue 1wk after leaving*]; *or* [mefloquine 250mg Q wk, *3wk before arrival, continue 4wk after leaving*]; *or* [doxycycline 100mg po QD, *start 2d before arrival, continue 4wk after leaving*].

Disease	Regimen
Mastitis	
Postpartum	Clindamycin; *or* 1st-gen ceph; *or* dicloxacillin; *or* cloxacillin; *or* oxacillin; *or* nafcillin; *or* methicillin. **Etiol:** *Staph. aureus.* Warm compresses/continued bilateral breast-feeding or pumping will hasten recovery.
Other	Clindamycin; *or* [metronidazole *and* (1st-gen ceph *or* oxacillin *or* dicloxacillin *or* nafcillin *or* methicillin *or* vancomycin)]; *or* amoxicillin clavulanate; *or* ampicillin/sulbactam. **Etiol:** *Staph. aureus, Bacteroides, Peptococcus.*
Mastoiditis	*Child/adult:* (2nd- or 3rd-gen ceph) *and* (gentamicin *or* ciprofloxacin *or* levofloxacin *or* gatifloxacin *or* moxifloxacin *or* ticarcillin/clavulanate *or* piperacillin/tazobactam. Surgical drainage often required for acute cases. Use fluoroquinolones only if ≥18y.o.*
Meningitis	Goal is antibiotics ASAP, then obtain CSF in 30min. If CT indicated before LP, give ABs, then CT, then LP.
Treatment	For suspected bacterial etiology with no CNS leak and no recent neurosurgical procedure, give with or just before 1st AB dose dexamethasone *adults only* 10mg IV, then 10mg IV Q 6h for 4d.
Infant <1mo.	[Ampicillin *and* (gentamicin *or* cefotaxime)]. **Etiol:** Group B or D *Strep., Enterobacteriaceae, Listeria, E. coli.*
Infant 1-3mo.	[(Ampicillin *or* vancomycin) *and* (cefotaxime *or* ceftriaxone)]. **Etiol:** *H. influenzae, Pneumococci, Meningococci, and same as infant <1mo. old.*
Child 3mo.-adult 50y.o.	[Vancomycin *and* (cefotaxime *or* ceftriaxone)]; *or* meropenem. *Base use of vancomycin on prevalence of drug-resistant S. pneumoniae.* **Etiol:** *Pneumococci, Meningococci, H. influenzae (now rare).*

TREATMENT OF SPECIFIC DISEASES *(continued)*

Disease	Regimen
Adult >50y.o. or medically complicated	[(Vancomycin 1g IV Q 6-12h) *and* (ceftriaxone 2g IV Q 12h *or* cefotaxime 2g IV Q 6h) *and* (ampicillin 2g IV Q 4h)]; *or* meropenem 1g IV Q 8h. **Etiol:** *Pneumococci; also: Enterobacteriaceae,H. influenzae, Listeria, Pseudomonas.*
HIV infection	**Etiol:** *Cryptococcus most common; also: TB, syphilis, aseptic HIV infection, Listeria monocytogenes, and same as seen in >50y.o.* *For cryptococcus:* Amphotericin 0.7-1.0 mg/kg/d IV, until afebrile and N, V, headache resolve, *then* fluconazole 400mg po QD to complete 8-10wk course, *then* fluconazole 100-200mg/d po as suppressive measure indefinitely.
Post neurosurg. procedure or craniospinal trauma	[(Vancomycin 1g IV Q 6-12h) *and* (ceftazidime 2g IV Q 8h.)]. *Vancomycin until known not to be MRSA. For Pseudomonas, add:* Tobramycin IV/intrathecal. **Etiol:** *Staph. aureus, Enterobacteriaceae, Pseudomonas, Pneumococci.*
Persistent CNS leak	*Child/adult:* Cefotaxime *or* ceftriaxone. **Etiol:** *Pneumococci.*
V-P or other CNS shunt	*Child:* Vancomycin 15 mg/kg IV Q 6h *and* (cefotaxime 50 mg/kg IV Q 6h *or* ceftriaxone 50 mg/kg Q 12h). *Adult:* Vancomycin *and* rifampin. *If gram-negative rods seen on Gram stain, add:* 3rd-gen ceph. *Shunt removal usually required for cure.* **Etiol:** *Staph. epidermidis, diphtheroids, Enterobacteriaceae.*

Prophylaxis

H. influenzae meningitis: *Child/adult:* Rifampin 20mg/kg (max 600mg) po QD for 4d. *Indications:* (1) all household contacts, regardless of age, in households with any incompletely vaccinated contact <48mo. old. *Household contact* = living with index pt (IP), or spent ≥4h with IP for 5 of 7d before dx of IP; (2) *single case* at child care locale/ nursery school if: (a) attended by unvaccinated or incompletely vaccinated child <2y.o. and children contact each other ≥25h/wk: treat all attendees, vaccinated or not; *or* (b) if ≥2 cases: treat all attendees and supervisory personnel, regardless of contact hours.

Disease	Regimen

Meningococcal meningitis: *Child/adult:* Rifampin 10mg/kg (max dose 600mg) po BID for 2d, **generally preferred;** *or* ceftriaxone 125mg (*child*) or 250mg IM (*adult*) single dose **preferred if preg;** *or* ciprofloxacin 500mg single dose *only if ≥18y.o.;* or azithromycin 500mg po single dose (*adults only*). *Indications:* (1) *all* household, child care, nursery school contacts; (2) contact with oral secretions through kissing or sharing food/drink; (3) **not** medical personnel, unless intimate contact such as intubation, suctioning, etc. Treat ASAP, preferably within 24h.

Myasthenia gravis
Diagnosis
(Tensilon test)

Child >1mo.: Edrophonium 0.04mg/kg (max 1mg if <34kg, 2mg if ≥34kg IV) over 15sec. If no response after 1min, may give 0.16mg/kg. *Max total dose:* 5mg if <34kg, 8mg if ≥34kg.
Adult: Obtain edrophonium 10mg in syringe. Give 2mg IV over 15-30sec. If no response in 45sec, give remaining 8mg IV over 30sec. *Positive test = objective improvement in contractility as well as subjective response.*

Myasthenic crisis
(undertreated)

Child: Neostigmine 0.01-0.04mg/kg SC/IM/IV Q 2-3h prn *or* pyridostigmine 2mg IM/IV Q 2-3h prn.
Adult: Neostigmine 0.5-2.5mg SC/IM/IV Q 4h.

Cholinergic crisis
(overtreated)

Child: Atropine 0.01-0.04mg/kg IV (max 0.5mg).
Adult: Atropine 0.5mg IV. *Supportive Rx also necessary. Sx: weakness, excessive sweating, salivation, lacrimation, small pupils, tachycardia, GI hyperactivity.*

Myocardial infarction

See coronary syndromes.

Needlestick protocol

HIV transmission rate = 0.3%; HBV rate = 10%. See p. 74 for Detroit Medical Center protocol to assess risk of exposure. If exposure warrants prophylaxis and source is known HIV-positive or has positive rapid HIV test, start lamivudine 150mg po BID *plus* zidovudine 300mg po BID *plus* [nelfinavir 1250mg po BID or indinavir 800mg po TID)] within 24-36h; best results if initiated within 1-2h and

(continued on following page)

TREATMENT OF SPECIFIC DISEASES *(continued)*

Disease	Regimen
Needlestick protocol *(cont'd)*	continued for 28d. If source is on antiretroviral medications, consult ID specialist for specific recommendations or call PEP-line (Postexposure Prophylaxis) at 1-800-448-4911; advice available 24h/day. Assess for HBV infectious status of source and vaccination status of exposed. If non-vaccinated or inadequate antibody response antiHbsAg titer ≤10 mIU/ml, give HBIG and HBV vaccine.
Neuroleptic malignant syndrome	*Child/adult:* Diazepam *or* lorazepam 5-15min IM/IV for sedation prn *and* bromocriptine 2.5-5mg po TID. Occurs 3-9d after starting or dosage increase of antipsychotic agent. Signs: hyperthermia, muscle rigidity, autonomic instability, altered MS.
Osteomyelitis *Newborn*	[(Nafcillin *or* methicillin *or* oxacillin *or* vancomycin) *and* 3rd-gen ceph]. **Etiol:** *Staph. aureus,* Enterobacteriaceae, Groups A and B *Strep.*
Child <4 years	[(Nafcillin *or* methicillin *or* oxacillin *or* vancomycin) *and* (3rd-gen ceph *or* amikacin *or* gentamicin *or* tobramycin)]. **Etiol:** *Streptococci, Staph. aureus.*
Child >4 years-adult	Nafcillin; *or* methicillin; *or* oxacillin; *or* 1st-gen ceph; *or* vancomycin; *or* (ciprofloxacin *only if >18y.o and* rifampin). **Etiol:** *Staph. aureus; Enterobacteriaceae and Streptococci are much less common.*
Hemodialysis or IVDU	[(Nafcillin *or* methicillin *or* oxacillin *or* vancomycin) *and* (ciprofloxacin *only if >18y.o.*)]. **Etiol:** *Staph. aureus, Pseudomonas.*
Puncture wound	Ciprofloxacin *only if ≥18y.o.; or* cefoperazone; *or* ceftazidime. **Etiol:** *Pseudomonas; Staph. aureus is much less common.*

See index for generic names of proprietary meds

Disease	Regimen
Post-op or post-trauma	[Nafcillin 2g Q 4h *and* ciprofloxacin 750mg IV/PO BID]; *or* [vancomycin *and* 3rd-gen ceph]. **Etiol:** *Staph. aureus, Enterobacteriaceae, Pseudomonas.*
Post-sternotomy	[Vancomycin 1g Q 12h IV *and* rifampin 600-900mg po QD]. **Etiol:** *Staph. epi.*
Sickle cell anemia	Ciprofloxacin *only if ≥18y.o.*; *or* 3rd-gen ceph. **Etiol:** *Salmonella.*
Vertebral	*Post laminectomy:* Nafcillin; *or* methicillin; *or* oxacillin; *or* vancomycin. **Etiol:** *Staph. aureus, Staph. epidermidis.* *Blood-borne:* [Ciprofloxacin *only if ≥18y.o. and* rifampin]; *or* ticarcillin/clavulanate; *or* [vancomycin *and* 3rd-gen ceph]; *or* imipenem. **Etiol:** *Staph. aureus, Enterobacteriaceae, P. aeruginosa, Candida.*

Otitis

Disease	Regimen
Bullous myringitis	*Child/adult:* Erythromycin; *or* azithromycin; *or* clarithromycin. *Dosing as for otitis media.* **Etiol:** *Mycoplasma pneumoniae, Chlamydia psittaci.*
Externa	*Child/adult:* [(Irrigation of canal, placement of Merocel wick if *severe edema* present) *and* (polymyxin B/neomycin/hydrocortisone [*Cortisporin*] 4 drops QID [use emulsion if TM perf.] *or* acetic acid 2% with hydrocortisone 4 drops QID *or* ofloxacin 0.3% 2 drops BID)]. *Remove wick in 5d.* **Etiol:** *Pseudomonas species, Enterobacteriaceae, Proteus species.*
Malignant (invasive with cellulitis surrounding canal)	*Child/adult:* Treat as for externa, add: imipenem; *or* meropenem; *or* ciprofloxacin *only if ≥18y.o.*; *or* cefoperazone; *or* ceftazidime; *or* ticarcillin; *or* [(ticarcillin/clavulanate *or* mezlocillin *or* piperacillin *or* piperacillin/tazobactam) *and* (amikacin *or* gentamicin *or* tobramycin)]. Strong association with DM; check BS. **Etiol:** *Pseudomonas species.*

TREATMENT OF SPECIFIC DISEASES *(continued)*

Disease	Regimen
Media	*Child:* [Amoxicillin 30mg/kg po TID **preferred initial treatment**]; *or* [amoxicillin/clavulanate 7-13mg/kg (max 500mg) po TID]; *or* [azithromycin 10mg/kg (max 500mg) po day 1, then 5mg/kg (max 250) po days 2-5] *or* [clarithromycin 7.5mg/kg (max 500mg) po BID]. *Adult:* [Amoxicillin 500mg po TID]; *or* [amoxicillin/clavulanate 875mg po BID]; *or* [azithromycin 500mg po day 1, then 250mg po days 2-5]; *or* [clarithromycin 500mg po BID]. *Rx child<2y.o. for 10d; child ≥2y.o.-adult for 5-7d.* **Etiol:** *S. pneumoniae, H. influenzae, M. catarrhalis.*

Pelvic inflammatory disease

Inpatient	*Admit if:* Dx unclear, possible surgical emergency, possible pelvic abscess, pregnant, adolescent pt, severe illness, patient cannot tolerate outpatient therapy, outpatient therapy has failed, patient cannot follow up in 72h, patient is HIV+. [(Cefoxitin 2g IV Q 6h *or* cefotetan 2g IV Q 12h *or* ampicillin/sulbactam 3g IV Q 6h) *and* doxycycline 100mg po/IV Q 12h]; *or* [(ofloxacin 400mg IV Q 12h *and* metronidazole 500mg IV Q 8h]; *or* [(gentamicin loading 2 mg/kg IM/IV, then gentamicin 1.5mg/kg IM/IV Q 8h) *and* (clindamycin 900mg IV Q 8h)]; *or* [ciprofloxacin 200mg IV Q 12h *and* metronidazole 500mg IV Q 8h *and* doxycycline 100mg po/IV Q 12h]. *Continue IV antibiotics for 48h after substantial clinical improvement, then start or continue* doxycycline 100mg po BID *to complete 14d of therapy.*

Disease	Regimen
Outpatient	[Ceftriaxone 250mg IM single dose *and* doxycycline 100mg po BID for 14d]; *or* [ofloxacin 400mg po BID *and* metronidazole 500mg po BID] for 14d]. **Etiol:** *N. gonorrhoea, C. trachomatis, Bacteroides species, Enterobacteriaceae, Strep. species.*
Pemphigus vulgaris	*Adult:* Prednisone 100-300mg po QD *with or without* (azathioprine 1mg/kg po QD *or* cyclophosphamide 1mg/kg po QD). *Potentially life-threatening; consult dermatology immediately.*
Peritonitis	
Bowel perforation	[Ampicillin *and* gentamicin *and* metronidazole]; *or* [(clindamycin *or* metronidazole) *and* (amikacin *or* gentamicin *or* tobramycin *or* aztreonam *or* piperacillin *or* mezlocillin *or* carbenicillin *or* ticarcillin *or* 2nd-/3rd-/4th-gen ceph *or* ciprofloxacin IV *only if ≥18y.o.* or ofloxacin *IV only if ≥18y.o.*)]; *or* cefoxitin; *or* cefotetan; *or* cefmetazole; *or* ticarcillin/clavulanate; *or* piperacillin/tazobactam; *or* ampicillin/sulbactam; *or* imipenem; *or* meropenem. **Etiol:** *Enterobacteriaceae, enterococci, Bacteroides, P. aeruginosa.*
CAPD-related	*Gram-pos orgs on Gram stain:* Vancomycin 30 mg/kg IP Q 5-7d. [*Diagnosis if >100 WBC/mm^3 with >50% PMNs. If severe, may require admission for IV antibiotics and catheter removal.*] *Gram-neg orgs on Gram stain:* (ceftazidime 1g IP in 1 exchange QD) *or* (aztreonam 3g IP load and 1g IP in 1 exchange QD).
Spontaneous bacterial	Cefotaxime; *or* ticarcillin/clavulanate; *or* piperacillin/tazobactam; *or* ampicillin/sulbactam; *or* ceftriaxone; *or* ofloxacin. **Etiol:** Enterobacteriaceae, *Staph. aureus, S. pneumoniae,* Group A *Strep.*

TREATMENT OF SPECIFIC DISEASES *(continued)*

Disease	Regimen
Pertussis	*Child:* (Erythromycin 10-12.5mg/kg in child, up to 500mg po/IV QID for 14d); *or* (TMP-SMX as trimeth 5mg/kg po Q 12h for 14d); *or* (clarithromycin 7.5-10mg/kg, max 500mg, po BID for 14d); *or* (azithromycin 10-12mg/kg, max 500mg, po QD for 7d). *Adult:* (Erythromycin 500mg po/IV for 14d *or* TMP-SMX 1 DS tab po Q 12h for 14d); *or* (clarithromycin 500mg po BID for 14d); *or* (azithromycin 500mg po QD for 7d). Obtain nasopharyngeal swab/aspirate for culture or PCR. *Treat with ABs and initiate DTP vacc. for acute illness and all close contacts.*
Pharyngitis	Consider monospot testing for Epstein-Barr virus for adolescents/young adults or for recurrent cases. For severe exudative pharyngitis of any etiology, dexamethasone 0.15mg/kg up to 10mg IM or po once may speed resolution of sx.
Diphtheria	*Child/adult:* [(PCN G 40,000U/kg IV Q 6h for 10-14d) *or* (erythromycin 20-25 mg/kg IV Q 12h for 10-14d) *and* (give antitoxin as soon as possible if dx suspected—obtain from CDC, phone 404-639-8200)]. *Suspect if pt not immunized or recent immigrant from endemic areas, esp. former Soviet Union.*
Gonococcal	See p. 110.
Group A Strep.	*Empirical treatment more cost-effective than culture.* *Child:* [Benzathine PCN 600,000U (<27 kg) or 1.2 MU (≥27 kg) IM]; *or* [PCN VK 250mg po TID for 10d]. **PCN is preferred, but if PCN allergic:** [Erythromycin 10-20 mg/kg/dose (max 500mg) po BID for 10d]; *or* [azithromycin 12 mg/kg (max 500mg) po QD for 5d]; *or* [clarithromycin 7.5 mg/kg po (max 500mg) BID for 10d]; or [2nd-gen ceph po for 4-6d].

See index for generic names of proprietary meds

Disease	Regimen
	Adult: [Benzathine PCN 1.2 MU IM once]; *or* [(PCN VK 250mg po TID) *or* (PCN VK 500mg po BID) for 10d]. **PCN is preferred, but if PCN allergic:** [azithromycin 500mg po on day 1, then 250mg po QD on days 2-5]; *or* [clarithromycin 250mg BID for 10d]; *or* [2nd- or 3rd-gen ceph po for 4-6d]; *or* [erythromycin 500mg po BID for 10d].
Ludwig angina	*Child/adult:* PCNG 60,000U/kg (max 4 MU) IV Q 4h; or clindamycin 10mg/kg (max 600mg) IV Q 6h.
Pneumocystis pneumoniae New-onset pneumonia – clinical AIDS or HIV+	*Start suppressive therapy after completing course.* *Child:* TMP/SMX (as trimeth) 5mg/kg (max 160mg) po/IV Q 6h for 14-21d **preferred;** *or* pentamidine 3-4mg/kg IV QD for 14-21d. *If >13y.o. and pO2 <70, add prednisone 40mg po BID for 5d, then 20mg po QD for 11d with first dose before initial anti-pneumocystis therapy. Although most believe younger hypoxic children would benefit from steroids, optimal dose and course not established.* *Adult:* **Mild disease (not acutely ill, pO2 >70, can take oral meds):** TMP/SMX 2 DS tabs po TID for 21d **preferred;** *or* [trimethoprim 5 mg/kg po Q 6h *and* dapsone 100mg po QD for 21d]; *or* [primaquine base 30mg po QD *and* clindamycin 450mg po or 600mg IV Q 8h for 21d]; *or* atovaquone 750mg po BID with meals for 21d. *Adult:* **Severe disease (acutely ill, pO2 <70, cannot take oral meds):** TMP/SMX (as trimeth) 5 mg/kg IV Q 8h for 21d **preferred;** *or* pentamidine 4 mg/kg IV QD for 21d; *or* [trimetrexate 45mg/m^2 IV QD for 21d *and* folinic acid 20mg po/IV Q 6h for 24d]. *Start prednisone 15-30min before above drugs at 40mg po BID for 5d, then 40mg po QD for 5d, then 20mg po QD for 11d.*

See index for generic names of proprietary meds

TREATMENT OF SPECIFIC DISEASES *(continued)*

Disease	Regimen
Chronic suppression	*Child:* TMP/SMX (as trimeth) 75mg/m^2 (max 80mg) po BID given every day or 3 times/wk **preferred;** *or* dapsone 1 mg/kg (max 100mg) po QD; *or* (*only if >5y.o.*) pentamidine 4 mg/kg IM Q 2-4wk.
	Adult: TMP/SMX 1 DS tab po 3 times/wk **preferred;** *or* dapsone 100mg po QD; *or* pentamidine 300mg in 6ml sterile water Q 4wk by Respirgard II nebulizer; *or* atovaquone 1500mg po QD; *or* (dapsone 200mg po QD *and* pyrimethamine 75mg po QD *and* folinic acid 25mg po QD).

Pneumonia	Assess mortality risk/need for hospitalization with clinical decision rule (pp. 21-22).
Child <1mo.	[(Ampicillin *or* nafcillin *or* vancomycin) *and* (gentamicin *or* cefotaxime)].
	Etiol: CMV, Rubella, HSV, Group B *Strep., Listeria,* coliforms, *Chlamydia.*
Child 1-3mo.	**Pneumonitis syndrome** (*cough, dyspnea, tachypnea, diffuse infiltrates, afebrile*): Erythromycin 10mg/kg IV Q 6h for 10-14d; *or* clarithromycin 7.5mg/kg po BID for 10-14d. *Most cases require admission.*
	Etiol: *C. trachomatis, RSV, other respiratory viruses, Bordetella.*
Child 1-24mo.	**Admitted but not ICU:** Cefuroxime 50mg/kg IV Q 8-12h.
	Admitted ICU: [Cefotaxime 67mg/kg Q 8h *and* erythromycin 10mg/kg IV Q 6h for 10-14d].
	Etiol: *S. pneumoniae, H. influenzae, Chlamydia, Mycoplasma, Staph. aureus.*
Child 3mo.-5y.o.	**Outpatient Rx:** Erythromycin 10mg/kg po QID; *or* clarithromycin 7.5mg/kg po BID.
	Admitted floor or ICU: [Cefuroxime 50mg/kg IV Q 8h *and* erythromycin 10mg/kg Q 6h].
	Etiol: *S. pneumoniae, Mycoplasma, Chlamydia.*

Disease	Regimen
Child 5-18y.o.	Clarithromycin; *or* azithromycin; *or* doxycycline; *or* erythromycin.
	Etiol: *Mycoplasma, respiratory viruses.*
Adult, influenza	Oseltamivir; *or* amantadine; *or* rimantadine. *Oseltamivir effective for influenza types A & B; amantadine and rimantadine effective only for influenza type A.*
Aspiration	*Child/adult:* Cefoxitin; *or* cefotetan; *or* [(clindamycin) *and* (gentamicin *or* amikacin *or* tobramycin)]; *or* [(ceftriaxone *or* cefotaxime) *and* (metronidazole]; *or* ampicillin/sulbactam; *or* piperacillin/ tazobactam.
Adult, community acquired	Assess mortality risk and need for hospitalization with clinical decision rule; see pp. 21-22.
	Outpt Rx: Azithromycin 500mg, then 250mg QD for 4d; *or* clarithromycin 500mg po BID; or clarithromycin ER 1g po QD; *or* amoxicillin/ clavulanate 875mg po QD; *or* 2nd- or 3rd-gen ceph; *or* levofloxacin; *or* moxifloxacin; *or* gatifloxacin; *or* ciprofloxacin.
	Admitted, non-ICU: Treat IV with ceftriaxone; *or* cefotaxime; *or* ceftizoxime; *or* cefepime; *or* [(ampicillin/sulbactam) *and* (azithromycin *or* clarithromycin *or* erythromycin)]; *or* levofloxacin; *or* moxifloxacin; *or* gatifloxacin; *or* ciprofloxacin.
	Admitted, ICU: Same as non-ICU for most pts; consider addition of vancomycin to cover resistant gram-positive organisms. *If critically ill:* [(Ceftriaxone *or* cefotaxime *or* ceftizoxime *or* cefepime *or* ampicillin/sulbactam) *and* (azithromycin *or* erythromycin) *and* (gentamicin *or* amikacin *or* tobramycin)].
	Etiol: ***Healthy:*** *Mycoplasma, Chlamydia pneumoniae,* viral. ***Smokers:*** *S. pneumoniae, H. influenzae, Moraxella.* ***Post-viral:*** *S. pneumoniae, Staph. aureus.* ***Alcoholic:*** *S. pneumoniae,* anaerobes, coliforms. ***IVDU:*** *S. pneumoniae.*

TREATMENT OF SPECIFIC DISEASES *(continued)*

Disease	Regimen
Adult, hospital acquired	Imipenem; *or* meropenem; or [(piperacillin/ tazobactam *or* ticarcillin/clavulanate *or* cefepime *or* ceftazidime) *and* (tobramycin)]. **Etiol: *Hospital acquired:*** *S. pneumoniae,* anaerobes, coliforms.
Adult, neutropenic	Same as for hospital acquired, but consider addition of amphotericin if persistent fever. **Etiol:** *As for community acq./hospitalized acq., add fungi.*
Prostatitis	Exercise caution when performing examination; manipulation of inflamed prostate/Foley cath can precipitate bacteremia. *Acute, outpt Rx:* [(TMP-SMX 1 DS tab po BID); *or* (ciprofloxacin 500mg po BID); *or* (norfloxacin 400mg po BID); *or* (ofloxacin 400mg po BID); *or* (levofloxacin 500mg po QD) for 30d]. *Acute, inpt or seriously ill:* [(Ampicillin 2 g IV Q 6h) *and* (gentamicin *or* tobramycin 5-7mg/kg IV QD until stable), then continue oral meds as above for 30d course]. *Chronic:* Consider dx if recurrent UTIs with same organism. Treat with a fluoroquinolone. Same dosing as for acute, often requires prolonged course up to 12wk. Consider dx if recurrent UTIs with same organism.
Pulmonary embolism	Use clinical decision rules (p. 20) to determine pre-test prob. of PE. If high prob., start anti-coagulation before imaging study. Determine d-dimer from 1st drawn blood to minimize false +.
Hemodynamically stable	Heparin 80U/kg IV bolus, then 18U/kg/h IV; or enoxaparin 1 mg/kg SC Q 12h or 1.5mg/kg SC QD; *or* tinzaparin 175 U/kg SC QD; *or* dalteparin 200U/kg SC QD or 100U/kg SC Q 12h). *Consider thrombolytics (below) if echo shows RV dysfunction.*

See index for generic names of proprietary meds

Disease	Regimen
Massive with hemodynamic instability/ persistent hypoxia	Alteplase 10mg IV bolus, then 90mg IV over 2h; *or* reteplase 10U IV over 2min, repeat dose in 30min; *or* streptokinase 250,000U IV over 30min, then infusion of 100,000U/h for 24h; *or* urokinase 4400U/kg IV over 10min, then infusion of 4400U/kg/h for 12h. Risk of intracranial hemorrhage ~1-2%. Hold anticoagulation during thrombolytic treatment; at completion, check PTT, start UFH or LMWH once PTT < 2.5x control.
Rabies prophylaxis	*Child/adult:* (HRIG 20IU/kg with ≥50% infiltrated at bite site and remainder IM) *and* (HDCV vaccine 1ml IM on days 0, 3, 7, 14, and 28). May be indicated for high-risk animals (bats, raccoons, skunks, foxes, coyotes, dogs in developing countries or along U.S.-Mexico border and feral cats). Avoid suture closure if extremity injury. Antibiotic prophylaxis should be given for 5d (see p. 43).
Rhabdomyolysis	*Adult:* Maintaining euvolemia is crucial. Administer 0.9% NS to maintain urine output 200-300cc/h. If CK >10,000U/L, consider infusion of sodium bicarbonate 1-2 amps (44 mEq/amp) in 1L 0.45% NS or D5W at 100cc/h, titrate to urinary pH >7. After fluid resuscitation, consider mannitol 1-2g/kg IV over 30min, repeat Q 4-6h prn.
Scabies	*Child/adult:* Permethrin 5% cream apply from neck down, wash off in 8-14h **preferred**; *or* ivermectin 200µg/kg po once); *or* [lindane 1% cream or lotion apply from neck down and wash off in 8-14h (do not use in children < 2y.o. or if extensive dermatitis)]. Eradication requires thorough cleaning or destruction of clothes, bedsheets. Reevaluate in 7d; consider re-treatment if sx persist.

TREATMENT OF SPECIFIC DISEASES (continued)

Disease	Regimen
Sepsis, unknown source	

Septic shock
Early goal-directed therapy with support of specific parameters (CVP 8-12mm Hg, MAP 65-90mm Hg, central venous O_2 saturation ScvO$_2$ ≥70%, Hct ≥30%) with crystalloid/colloid sltns, vasoactive agents, PRBCs is the most cost-effective, life-saving approach. *If multi-organ system failure: Adult:* Consider drotrecogin (activated Protein C) 24µg/kg/h for 96h (cost = $8K).

Child <1mo. old
[Ampicillin *and* (cefotaxime *or* ceftriaxone *or* amikacin *or* gentamicin *or* tobramycin)].
Etiol: Group B *Strep., E. coli, Klebsiella, Enterobacter, Staph. aureus, H. influenzae.*

Child >1mo. old, not immunocompromised
Cefotaxime; *or* ceftriaxone; *or* cefuroxime.
Etiol: *H. influenzae, S. pneumoniae, meningococci, Staph. aureus.*

Adult, not immunocompromised
Ticarcillin/clavulanate; *or* piperacillin/tazobactam; *or* imipenem; *or* meropenem; *or* [3rd-gen ceph *and* (metronidazole *or* clindamycin)]; *or* [clindamycin *and only if >18y.o* (ciprofloxacin *or* ofloxacin)].
Etiol: *Gram-positive cocci, gram-negative aerobic bacilli, anaerobes.*

Neutropenia (PMN <500/mm3)
Child/adult: Ceftazidime; *or* imipenem; *or* cefepime *or* [(carbenicillin *or* ticarcillin *or* piperacillin *or* mezlocillin *or* ceftazidime *or* cefoperazone) *and* (amikacin *or* gentamicin *or* tobramycin)]. *Add* vancomycin *if catheter implicated, if gram-positive organisms cultured, if hypotensive, if ongoing fluoroquinolone prophylaxis, or if known to be colonized by MRSA.*
Etiol: *Enterobacteriaceae, Pseudomonas, Staph. aureus or epidermidis, Viridans strep.*

See index for generic names of proprietary meds

Disease	Regimen
Splenectomized	*Child/adult:* Cefotaxime; *or* ceftriaxone. **Etiol:** *S. pneumoniae, H. influenzae, meningococci.*
IV drug use	*Adult:* [(Methicillin *or* nafcillin *or* oxacillin *or* vancomycin) *and* (amikacin *or* gentamicin *or* tobramycin)]. **Etiol:** *Staph. aureus; gram-negative bacilli less common.*
Sexual assault	*General:* Provide appropriate counseling/psychosocial support. Evidence collection/storage is essential. Obtain preg. test, baseline HIV, HBV RPR; repeat at 6, 12, 24wk after incident. *STD prophylaxis:* Ceftriaxone 125mg IM once *and* metronidazole 2g po once *and* (azithromycin 1g po once **prefered if preg** *or* doxycycline 100mg po BID for 7d). *Preg. prophylaxis:* [(Ovral 2 tabs po *or* Lo-Ovral 4 tabs po) *and* repeat dose in 12h with concurrent antiemetic, e.g., promethazine/prochlorperazine for 1d]. *HBV prophylaxis:* Vaccine only (see p. 204) if unimmunized; if immunized, assess antibody response and treat prn (see p. 112 for guidelines). *HIV prophylaxis:* High risk if multiple assailants, mucosal lesions present, or vaginal, oral, anal penetration/ trauma. If high risk, offer [(lamivudine 150mg po BID) *and* (zidovudine 300mg po BID) *and* (nelfinavir 1250mg po BID *or* indinavir 800mg po TID) and arrange F/U in 3-7d]. If low risk, or HIV treatment declined, arrange F/U in 1-2wk.
Sinusitis	*Treat all children/adults with decongestants:* [(Phenylephrine *or* oxymetazoline nasal spray) *and/or* (pseudoephedrine po) *and/or steroid nasal sprays* (beclomethasone *or* fluticasone *or* mometasone *or* budesonide)]. Indications for 10d AB course: (1) Failure of oral and/or nasal decongestants in 3-5d with unilateral purulent nasal discharge and sinus pain, (2) severe disease on initial presentation (fever/pain).

(continued on following page)

See index for generic names of proprietary meds

TREATMENT OF SPECIFIC DISEASES *(continued)*

Disease	Regimen
Sinusitis *(cont'd)*	*Antibiotics child/adult:* [Amoxicillin 30mg/kg po TID]; *or* [amoxicillin/clavulanate 7-13mg/kg (max 500mg) po TID]; *or* [azithromycin 10mg/kg (max 500mg) po day 1, then 5mg/kg (max 250mg) po days 2-5] *or* [clarithromycin 7.5mg/kg (max 500mg) po BID]. *Antibiotics for treatment failure:* Amoxicillin/ clavulanate; *or* 2nd- or 3rd-gen ceph po.
Spinal cord injury, acute	*Acute trauma, new cord deficit:* Methylprednisolone 30 mg/kg IV over 15min, then 45min later start infusion at 5.4 mg/kg/h for 23h if treatment starts ≤3h after injury and for 47h if treatment begins >3h after injury.
Staphylococcal scalded skin syndrome	*Child/adult:* [(Fluid support IV) *and* (nafcillin 25-30 mg/kg, max 3g, IV Q 6h) *or* (oxacillin 37.5 mg/kg, max 2g, IV Q 6h)].
Status epilepticus	*Child >1mo.:* Diazepam 0.25mg/kg (max 5mg) IV Q 15min prn; *or* lorazepam 0.05mg/kg (max 4mg) IV Q 15min prn. *If unsuccessful:* Phenobarbital 15-20mg/kg IV at max rate of 1mg/kg/min; *or* phenytoin 15-20mg/kg IV at max rate 1mg/kg/min; *or* fosphenytoin 15-20PE (phenytoin equivalent)/kg IM or IV at max rate 3PE/kg/min (absolute max 150PE/min). *If seizures persist:* Switch from phenobarb to phenytoin/fosphenytoin or vice versa. *If seizures still persist:* Consider general anesthesia. *Adult:* Lorazepam 2mg/min IV up to 0.1mg/kg; *or* diazepam 5mg IV Q 5min prn up to 20mg max. *At the same time, load with:* Phenytoin 18mg/kg at max rate 50mg/min; *or* fosphenytoin 18PE/kg IM or IV at 150PE/min. *If seizures persist:* Add phenobarbital 17mg/kg at ≤100mg/min. *If still seizing:* Re-bolus with phenobarbital 10mg/kg IV at ≤100mg/min. *If*

(continued on following page)

See index for generic names of proprietary meds

Disease	Regimen
	seizures still persist: Consider general anesthesia with pentobarbital 10-15mg/kg IV over 1h, then infusion at 1-3mg/kg/h; *or* propofol 1- 2mg/kg IV, then infusion at 1-15mg/kg/h.
	In all cases: Obtain rapid glucose, ABGs for acid-base status. Protect airway.
Stroke	See pp. 99-100.
Syphilis	
<1yr duration (primary or early latent)	*Child:* Benzathine PCN G 50,000U/kg (max 2.4 million U) single dose IM.
	Adult: Benzathine PCN G 2.4MU IM **preferred;** *or* [ceftriaxone as: 125mg IM QD for 10d *or* 250mg IM QOD for 5 doses *or* 1000mg IM QOD for 4 doses]; *or* doxycycline 100mg po BID for 14d; *or* tetracycline 500mg po QID for 14d.
1yr duration (late latent, cardiovascular, late benign)	*Child:* Benzathine PCN G 50,000U/kg (max 2.4MU) IM Q wk for 3 doses.
	Adult: Benthazine PCN 2.4 million U IM Q wk for 3 doses **preferred;** *or* doxycycline 100mg po BID for 4wk; *or* tetracycline 500mg po QID for 4wk.
Neurosyphilis	*Child:* Aqueous PCN G 50,000U/kg (max 2 million U) IV Q 6h for 10-14d.
	Adult: Aqueous PCN G 2-4 million U IV Q 4h for 10d **preferred;** *or* [procaine PCN 2.4 million U IM QD *and* probenecid 500mg po QID for 10d]. If *HIV+,* use IV regimen.
Temporal arteritis	*Adult:* ESR usually >80; definitive diagnosis by temporal artery bx; admit if neuro or visual sx. Prednisone 40-60mg po QD for 1mo., then taper.
Tinea	†*Griseofulvin doses here are given for "microsize" preparation–see p. 203.*

TREATMENT OF SPECIFIC DISEASES *(continued)*

Disease	Regimen
Capitis	*Child >2y.o.:* Griseofulvin† 10-20mg/kg (max 1000mg) po QD for 4-6wk; *or* ketoconazole 3.3-6.6mg/kg (max 200mg) po QD for 4wk. *Adult:* Terbinafine 250mg po QD for 2-8wk (depending on species); *or* ketoconazole 200mg po QD for 4wk.
Corporis	*Child/adult:* Topical miconazole *or* clotrimazole TID for 2–4wk. If one of these is unsuccessful, consider ketoconazole 200mg po QD for at least 4wk for adults or griseofulvin for children.
Cruris or pedis	*Child/adult:* Topical miconazole *or* clotrimazole BID for 2-4wk.
Unguium (onychomycosis)	*Child:* Terbinafine 67.5mg (*<20kg*) *or* 125mg (*20-40kg*) *or* 250mg (*>40kg*) for 6wk (**fingernails**) or 12wk (**toenails**). Adult: Terbinafine 250mg po QD for 6wk (**fingernails**) or 12wk (**toenails**); *or* itraconazole 200mg po QD for 3mo.; *or* fluconazole 150-300mg po Q wk for 3-6mo. (**fingernails**) or 6-12mo. (**toenails**).
Versicolor	*Child:* Topical ketoconazole for 2wk; *or* 2.5% selenium sulfide lotion QD for 7d. *Adult:* Ketoconazole 400mg po as a single dose.
Toxoplasmosis *Chorioretinitis, meningitis*	*Child:* [Pyrimethamine 1 mg/kg (max 100mg) po BID on day 1, then 1 mg/kg (max 25mg) po QD *and* sulfadiazine 25 mg/kg (max 2g) po QID *and* folinic acid 5-10mg po QD]. *Adult:* [Pyrimethamine 100mg po on day 1, then 25mg po QD *and* sulfadiazine 1-2g po QID *and* folinic acid 10-15mg po QD]. *For chorioretinitis, add prednisone 0.5mg/kg po BID until vision improves. Treat for 1-2wk after sx resolve. Dose folinic acid by following CBC & continue for 1wk after finishing pyrimethamine.*

See index for generic names of proprietary meds

Disease	Regimen
Cerebral	*Child:* Same dosages as for meningitis above.
	Adult: [Pyrimethamine 200mg po on day 1, then 75-100mg po QD, *and* (sulfadiazine 1.0-1.5g po QID *or* clindamycin 600mg po/IV Q 6h *or* clarithromycin 1g po BID *or* azithromycin 1.2-1.5g po QD *or* dapsone 100mg po QD) *and* folinic acid 10-15mg po QD]. *Sulfadiazine is* **preferred.** *Treat for 3-6wk, then begin suppressive Rx.*
Primary prophy-laxis in AIDS patients	*Child:* Trimeth 75mg/sulfa 375mg/m² po BID; *or* [dapsone 2mg/kg (max 25mg) po QD *and* pyrimethamine 1mg/kg (max 50mg) po QD *and* leucovorin 5mg po every 3d].
	Adult: TMP/SMX SS or DS 1 po QD; *or* [dapsone 50mg po QD *and* pyrimethamine 50mg po Q wk *and* folinic acid 25mg po Q wk].
Suppression after acute treatment of cerebral toxoplasmosis	*Child:* [Pyrimethamine 1mg/kg (max 50mg) po QD *and* sulfadiazine 25mg/kg (max 2g) po QID *and* folinic acid 5-10mg po QD].
	Adult: [Pyrimethamine 25-50mg po QD *and* folinic acid 10-25mg po QD *and* (sulfadiazine 0.5-1.0g po QID *or* clindamycin 300-450mg po TID)].

Transfusion reaction

Urticarial	*Sx:* Urticaria.
	Rx: Stop transfusion, give diphenhydramine 50mg IVP. If sx resolve, may re-start transfusion, using same blood.
Febrile	*Sx:* Fever, rigors.
	Rx: Stop transfusion, recheck blood ID, return blood to blood bank, blood cultures, antipyretics.
Non-hemolytic	*Sx:* Agitation, dyspnea, headache, malaise.
	Rx: Stop transfusion, recheck blood ID, return blood to blood bank, blood cultures. Obtain U/A, CBC, bilirubin, LDH, and haptoglobin. *Prompt response may prevent hemolysis.*

See index for generic names of proprietary meds

TREATMENT OF SPECIFIC DISEASES *(continued)*

Disease	Regimen
Hemolytic	***Sx:*** Agitation, dyspnea, headache, malaise, flank and/or infusion site pain, chest pain, hematuria, hemorrhage at venipuncture sites.
	Rx: Stop transfusion and return blood to blood bank, start dopamine 5µg/kg/min (renal dose). Obtain U/A, CBC, PT, PTT, fibrin D-dimer, LDH, bilirubin, haptoglobin.
Anaphylactic	***Sx:*** Anxiety, chest pain, urticaria, wheezing, shock.
	Rx: Stop transfusion and treat as for anaphylaxis (p. xxx). *Obtain same labs as for hemolytic reaction.*

Unstable angina	See p. 102.
Urethritis, non-gonoccocal	See p. 101.

Urinary tract infection	
Cystitis, uncomplicated	*Child:* Hospitalize if <3 mo. old. Amoxicillin; *or* amoxicillin/clavulanate; *or* TMP-SMX; *or* cephalexin; *or* cefixime. *Treat for 7d. Adult:* TMP-SMX 1 DS tab po BID for 3d appropriate for most cases. *Where E. coli R rates >20%:* For 3d norfloxacin *or* ciprofloxacin *or* levofloxacin *or* lomefloxacin *or* gatifloxacin. *If DM, prolonged sx, recurrence, diaphragm use, male, or age >65y.o.:* Use same ABs, but for 7d.
Pregnant	*Adult:* Amoxicillin 500mg po TID; *or* nitrofurantoin; *or* cefpodoxime. *Treat bacteriuria even if no sx. Treat for 7d.*
Pyelonephritis	*Usually women 18-40 y.o. with fever >102°F, CVA tenderness. Treat for at least 14d*
Pyelonephritis, outpatient	Consider OP only for stable nonpregnant pts who tolerate po and have adequate F/U. Treat for 14d.

Disease	Regimen
Pyelonephritis, inpatient IV	*Child:* Amoxicillin/clavulanate **preferred**; *or* TMP-SMX; *or* cephalexin. *Adult:* Same ABs as cystitis for 14d. *Child/adult:* (Gentamicin *and* ampicillin); *or* 3rd-gen ceph; *or* ampicillin/sulbactam; *or* piperacillin/tazobactam; *or* TMP-SMX; *or* (*only if ≥18y.o.:* Ciprofloxacin *or* levofloxacin *or* ofloxacin *or* gatifloxacin). *Pregnant:* (Gentamicin *and* ampicillin); *or* 3rd-gen ceph; *or* ampicillin/ sulbactam; *or* piperacillin/tazobactam.

Vaginitis

Bacterial vaginosis	*Not pregnant:* Metronidazole 500mg po BID for 7d **preferred;** *or* clindamycin cream 2% 1 full applicator intravaginally hs for 7d **preferred;** *or* metronidazole gel 0.75% 1 full applicator intravaginally BID for 5d **preferred;** *or* metronidazole 2g po single dose; *or* clindamycin 300mg po BID for 7d. *Pregnant:* Metronidazole 250mg po TID for 7d **preferred;** *or* metronidazole 2g po single dose; *or* clindamycin 300mg po BID for 7d. *If no hx of pre-term labor or PROM, may also use* metronidazole gel 0.75%, 1 full applicator intravaginally BID for 5d. *Bacterial vaginosis is associated with premature labor/PROM. Diagnose if three of these found: homogeneous, white non-inflammatory discharge adherent to vaginal walls; clue cells by micro; vaginal fluid pH >4.5; fishy odor to vaginal discharge sample before or after 10% KOH. Treat sexual partners only if balanitis present.*
Candida/yeast	Fluconazole 150mg po single dose; *or* butoconazole 2% cream; *or* clotrimazole 1% cream *or* clotrimazole vag tabs; *or* miconazole vag supp; *or* tioconazole 6.5% ointment; *or* terconazole 0.8% cream; *or* terconazole vag supp.

TREATMENT OF SPECIFIC DISEASES *(continued)*

Disease	Regimen
Trichomonas	*Mild-moderate: treat single dose; severe or complicated cases, or preg: treat for 3-7d.* *Child:* Metronidazole 40 mg/kg (max 2g) po single dose; *or* metronidazole 5 mg/kg (max 333mg) po TID for 7d. *Adult:* Metronidazole 2g po single dose; *or* metronidazole 500mg po BID for 7d. *If pregnant, use metronidazole 2g single-dose regimen above. Treat sexual partners. If single-dose therapy fails, try BID 7d regimen given above. For repeated failures:* Metronidazole 2g po QD for 3-5d.

Varicella/Zoster
  Chickenpox

Normal host	*Child 2-12y.o.:* Acyclovir 20mg/kg (max 800mg) po QID for 5d. *Child >12y.o.-adult:* Acyclovir 800mg po QID for 5d *or* 10mg/kg IV Q 8h for 5d. *Treat if: underlying skin/lung problem; on salicylates or steroids; clinically ill; >12y.o.; pneumonia present; pregnant; or if otherwise at risk for mod-severe chickenpox.*
Immunocomp or 3rd trimester preg	*Child/adult:* Acyclovir 10-12mg/kg IV Q 8h for 7-10d.
Post-herpetic neuralgia	*Adult:* Amitriptyline 12.5-25mg po QD, titrate to 150mg as needed; *or* carbamazepine 200mg po QD, titrate to 1200mg as needed; *or* gabapentin 300mg po TID, titrate to 1200mg po TID as needed).

  Zoster

Normal host (or mild case, immunocomp. pt)	*Child 12y.o.-adult:* Acyclovir 800mg po 5 times a day for 7d; *or* famciclovir 500mg po Q 8h for 7d; *or* valacyclovir 1000mg po TID for 7d. *If >50y.o. consider prednisone 30mg po BID for 7d, then 15mg po BID for 7d, then 7.5mg po BID for 7d.*

See index for generic names of proprietary meds

Disease	Regimen
Immunocomp./ severe case (>1 dermatome, trigeminal nerve involved, dissem. zoster)	*Child/adult:* Acyclovir 10-12mg/kg IV Q 8h for 7-14d. *Reduce to 7.5mg/kg for older patients or if renal insufficiency is present.*

Venous thrombosis, deep

Routine treatment

Child: Heparin 50U/kg IV, then infusion at 10-25U/kg/h *or* dalteparin 200U/kg SC QD or 100U/kg SC Q 12h).

Adult: Heparin 80U/kg IV, then infusion at 18U/kg/h; *or* enoxaparin 1mg/kg SC Q 12h; *or* tinzaparin 175U/kg SC QD. *Continue for 5-7d.* Start *Coumadin* 5mg on day 1 or 2. Discharge patient when INR >2, aim for INR 2-3. Continue *Coumadin* for at least 3mo. and up to lifetime, depending on risk factors.

Massive ileofemoral vein thrombosis

Child: Streptokinase 3500-4500U/kg IV over 30min, then 1000-1500U/kg/h for 24-48h.

Adult: Alteplase 100mg IV over 2h; *or* reteplase 10U IV over 2min, repeat dose in 30min; *or* streptokinase 250,000U IV, then 100,000U/h IV infusion for 24h. *Start heparin with thrombolytic agent: Adult:* 500-1000U/h.

Prophylaxis

Pre-op or bedridden: Heparin 70-125U/kg SC Q 12h; *or* enoxaparin 30-50mg SC Q 12h; *or* dalteparin 2500U SC QD; *or* tinzaparin 50U/kg SC QD.

von Willebrand's disease

See p. 79.

Worm infestations

Hookworm (Ancylostoma duodenale, Necator americanus)

Child/adult: Albendazole 400mg po single dose; *or* mebendazole 100mg po BID for 3d **preferred;** *or* pyrantel pamoate 11mg/kg (max 1g) po QD for 3d.

TREATMENT OF SPECIFIC DISEASES *(continued)*

Disease	Regimen
Pinworm (Enterobius vermicularis)	*Child/adult:* Albendazole 400mg po; *or* mebendazole 100mg po; *or* pyrantel pamoate 11mg/kg (max 1g) po. *For all of these regimens, repeat dose in 2wk; repeat pyrantel pamoate Q 2wk twice.*
Roundworm (Ascaris lumbricoides)	*Child/adult:* Albendazole 400mg po single dose; *or* mebendazole 100mg po BID for 3d; *or* pyrantel pamoate 11mg/kg (max 1g) po single dose.
Tapeworm	*Child/adult:* Praziquantel 10mg/kg po single dose.
*(Taenia saginata – **beef;** Diphyllobothrium lathium – **fish;** Taenia solium – **pork**)*	
Whipworm (Trichuris trichiura)	*Child/adult:* Albendazole 400mg po single dose; *or* mebendazole 100mg po BID for 3d.

See index for generic names of proprietary meds

This chapter consists of a table that lists drugs alphabetically by generic name, with the proprietary name(s) following in parentheses. The various preparations are listed for each drug, and dosing for each preparation is also listed. Pediatric doses are given when available. The final column of the table provides annotations related to pregnancy risk. A key to the abbreviations in this column is listed below.

Key to special annotations related to pregnancy risk:
2 = if used in 2nd trimester.
3 = if used in 3rd trimester.
2–3 = if used in 2nd or 3rd trimester.
*If used for prolonged periods or high doses at term.
§ If dosed above recommended requirement/d.
(Htn) = If used in pregnancy-induced HTN.

FDA Pregnancy Risk Categories:
A = Controlled studies in women fail to demonstrate a risk to the fetus in the first trimester (and there is no evidence of a risk in later trimesters), and the possibility of fetal harm appears remote.
B = Either animal-reproduction studies have not demonstrated a fetal risk but there are no controlled studies in pregnant women or animal-reproduction studies have shown an adverse effect (other than a decrease in fertility) that was not confirmed in controlled studies in women in the first trimester (and there is no evidence of a risk in later trimesters).
C = Either studies in animals have revealed adverse effects on the fetus (teratogenic or embryocidal or other) and there are no controlled studies in women or studies in women and animals are not available. Drugs should be given only if the potential benefit justifies the potential risk to the fetus.
D = There is positive evidence of human fetal risk, but the benefits from use in pregnant women may be acceptable despite the risk (e.g., if the drug is needed in a life-threatening situation or for a serious disease for which safer drugs cannot be used or are ineffective).
X = Studies in animals or human beings have demonstrated fetal abnormalities, or there is evidence of fetal risk in human experience, or both, and the risk from the use of the drug in pregnant women clearly outweighs any possible benefit. The drug is contraindicated in women who are or may become pregnant.

Medication	Preparation	Dosing	Pregnancy Risk
Abacavir (*Ziagen*)	*Liquid:* 20mg/ml *Tab:* 300mg	*Child 3mo.-16y.o.:* 8mg/kg po BID. *Child 16y.o.-adult:* 300mg po BID.	C
Abciximab (*ReoPro*)	*Inj:* 2mg/ml	*Adult:* give 0.25mg/kg bolus IV 10-60min before angioplasty, then 0.125µg/kg/min (max 10µg/min) for 12h.	C
Acarbose (*Precose*)	*Tab:* 25, 50, 100mg	**DM:** *Adult:* 25-100mg po TID. *If <60kg, max dose 150mg/d.*	B
Acebutolol (*Sectral*)	*Cap:* 200, 400mg	*Adult:* **HTN:** 400-800mg QD or divided BID, max 1200mg divided BID. **Ventricular arrhythmias:** start 200mg BID maintenance usually 600-1200mg/d.	B,D2-3
Acetaminophen (*Tylenol*)	*Drops:* 80mg/0.8ml *Liquid:* 80, 120, 160, 325mg/5ml, 500mg/15ml *Tab:* 80, 160mg (*both chew*); 325, 500, 650mg *ER Tab:* 650mg *Supp:* 80, 120, 325, 650mg	*Child:* 10-15mg/kg Q 4-6h, max 5 doses/d. *Adult:* 325-650mg Q 4-6h or 1000mg Q 6-8h. *ER-tab:* 650-1300mg Q 8h, max dose 4g/d.	B

See index for proprietary names of generic meds

Drug	Forms	Dosage	Preg
Acetaminophen/ codeine *(Tylenol with Codeine No. 2, No. 3, No. 4)*	*Liquid:* Acet 120mg/Codeine 12mg per 5ml *Tab:* Acet 300mg/Codeine 15, 30, or 60mg	*Child:* 0.5-1.0mg codeine/kg Q 4-6h. *Adult:* as codeine, 15-60mg Q 4-6h.	NR
Acetaminophen/ oxycodone *(Roxicet, Percocet, Tylox)*	*Tab:* Acet 325mg/Oxy 2.5mg, Acet 325mg/Oxy 5mg, Acet 325mg/Oxy 7.5mg, Acet 325mg/Oxy 10mg, Acet 500mg/Oxy 7.5mg, Acet 650mg/Oxy 10mg *Liquid:* Acet 325mg/Oxy 5mg per 5ml	*Adult:* 325-650mg APAP/2.5-10mg Q 6h.	NR
Acetazolamide *(Diamox, AK-Zol)*	*Tab:* 125, 250mg *Tab (LA):* 500mg *Inj:* 500mg/5ml	***Glaucoma:* PO:** *Child:* 2-7.5mg/kg Q 8h. *Adult:* 250-1000mg/d divided Q 6h. **IV:** *Child:* 5-10mg/kg Q 6h. *Adult:* 250mg IV Q 4h. *Max* 1g/*d.* **Tab (LA):** 500mg BID. **CHF:** 5mg/kg (*child*) or 250-375mg (*adult*) po/IV QD.	C
Acetohexamide *(Dymelor)*	*Tab:* 250, 500mg	*Adult:* 250-1500mg QD or divided BID.	C

Medication	Preparation	Dosing	Pregnancy Risk
Acetylcysteine (*Mucomyst, Acetadote*)	*Liquid*: (Mucomyst): 10%, 20% *Inj*: (Acetadote): 20% in 30ml	***Acetaminophen OD: PO:*** Mucomyst 140mg/kg, then 70mg/kg Q 4h for 17 doses.	B
Acyclovir (*Zovirax*)	*Liquid*: 200mg/5ml *Tab*: 400, 800mg *Cap*: 200mg *Ointment*: 5% *Inj*: 500, 1000mg/vial	***Herpes simplex:*** see pp. 114-115. ***Varicella:*** see pp. 142-143.	B
Adefovir (*Hepsera*)	*Tab*: 10mg	*Adult:* ***Chronic hepatitis B:*** 10mg QD.	C
Adenosine (*Adenocard*)	*Inj*: 6mg/2ml	*Child:* 0.05-0.1mg/kg IV rapidly; if necessary, may repeat; max total 0.25mg/kg or 30mg. *Adult:* 6mg IV rapidly, repeat 12mg IV Q 2min max 2 doses as necessary.	C
Albendazole (*Albenza*)	*Tab*: 200mg	***Worms:*** *see pp. 143-144.*	C
Albumin	*Inj*: 5% in 50, 250, 500, 1000ml; 25% in 20, 50, 100ml	***Hypovolemia:*** *Child:* 1g/kg (max 25g) IV over 30-120min. *Adult:* 25g IV.	C

See index for proprietary names of generic meds

Drug	Forms	Dosing	Preg
Albuterol (*Proventil*, *Ventolin*)	*Liquid:* 2mg/5ml *Tab:* 2, 4mg *Tab (SR):* 4, 8mg *Inhaler:* 90μg/puff *Inhalation sltn:* unit dose 2.5mg/3ml, 5mg/ml *Rotacap:* 200μg	**PO:** *Child <6y.o.:* 0.1mg/kg TID, max 2mg/dose. *Child 6-11y.o.:* 2mg TID-QID or 4mg SR tab BID. *Child >12y.o.-adult:* 2-4mg TID-QID or 1-2 SR tabs BID, max 32mg/d. **Inhaler:** *Child/adult:* 1-2 puffs Q 4-6h prn. **Nebulizer:** *Child:* 0.10-0.15mg/kg (max 5mg) in 2ml NS Q 4h. *Adult:* 2.5-5.0mg TID-QID. **Rotacaps:** *Child >4y.o.-adult:* 200μg Q 4-6h via Rotahaler.	C
Albuterol/ ipratropium (*Combivent*)	*Inhaler:* Alb 10μg/Ipra 1μg per puff *Inhalation sltn:* Alb 3mg/Ipra 0.5mg per 3ml	*Adult:* 2 puffs from inhaler QID or 1 neb from inhalation sltn QID	C
Alendronate (*Fosamax*)	*Tab:* 5, 10, 35, 40, 70mg	***Osteoporosis prevention:*** *Adult:* 5mg QD or 35mg Q week. ***Osteoporosis treatment:*** *Adult:* 10mg QD or 70mg Q week. ***Paget's:*** *Adult:* 40mg QD.	C
Alfuzosin (*Uroxatral*)	*Tab:* 10mg	*Adult:* **BPH:** 10mg QD after meal.	B
Allopurinol (*Zyloprim*)	*Tab:* 100, 200, 300mg	*Child:* 10mg/kg/d divided TID-QID, max 600mg/d. *Adult:* 100-800mg/d QD or in divided doses.	C

Medication	Preparation	Dosing	Pregnancy Risk
Almotriptan (*Axert*)	*Tab:* 6.25, 12.5mg	*Adult:* 6.25-12.5mg may repeat in 2h; max 2 doses/24h.	C
Alprazolam (*Xanax*)	*Tab:* 0.25, 0.5, 1, 2mg *Sltn:* 0.5mg/5ml; 1mg/ml	*Adult:* 0.25-1.0mg TID. *Start elderly, debilitated or chronically ill patients with low doses.*	D
Alteplase (*Activase*)	*Inj:* 1mg/ml in 50, 100ml vials	*PE: Adult:* 100mg IV over 120min. *Acute MI: Adult:* 15mg IVP, then 0.75mg/kg (max 50mg) over 30min, then 0.5mg/kg (max 35mg) over 60min. *Stroke:* see p. 99.	C
Aluminum hydroxide (*ALternaGEL, Alu-Cap, Alu-Tab, Amphojel*)	*Liquid:* 320, 450, 600, 675mg/5ml *Cap:* 400, 500mg *Tab:* 300, 600mg	*Child/adult: Liquid:* 500-1600mg (5-15ml) after meals and hs. *Tab:* 300-600mg; chew before swallowing with milk or water after meals and hs. *Cap:* 1-3 po after meals and hs. *Hyperphosphatemia in chronic renal failure: Child:* 50-150mg/kg/d divided Q 4-6h. *Adult:* 500-1800mg 3-6 times/d.	B
Amantadine (*Symmetrel*)	*Cap:* 100mg *Liquid:* 50mg/5ml	*Influenza A: Child 1-9y.o.:* 2.2-4.4mg/kg BID, max 150mg/d. *Child >9y.o.-adult:* 200mg/d QD or divided BID. *Most effective if started within 2d of sx; continue for 1-2d after sx resolve.* *Parkinson's: Adult:* 100mg BID; if seriously ill or receiving other anti-Parkinsonian drugs, 100mg QD for at least 1wk, then 100mg BID as needed.	C

See index for proprietary names of generic meds

Drug	Forms	Dosage	
Ambenonium (*Mytelase*)	*Tab:* 10mg	***Myasthenia gravis:*** 5-25mg TID-QID, max 200 mg/d.	C
Amikacin (*Amikin*)	*Inj:* 50, 250mg/ml	**IM/IV:** *Child <7d:* initial dose 10mg/kg, then 7.5 mg/kg Q 12h. *Child >7d-adult:* 15mg/kg/d divided Q 8-12h, max 1.5g/d. *Alternate QD dosing (adult only):* 15-20mg/kg IV only.	D
Amiloride (*Midamor*)	*Tab:* 5mg	*Child:* 0.625mg/kg QD. *Adult:* 5-20mg QD.	B
Amiloride/HCTZ (*Moduretic*)	*Tab:* Amiloride 5mg/HCTZ 50mg *Liquid:* 250mg, 1.25gm/ml	*Adult:* 1-2 tabs QD.	B
Aminocaproic acid (*Amicar*)	*Liquid:* 250mg, 1.25g/ml *Tab:* 500mg *Inj:* 250mg/ml	*Child:* 100mg/kg po/IV load, then 33.3mg/kg/h, max 18 g/m² /d. *Adult:* 4-5g IV load over 1h, then 1g/h infusion for 8h; or 5g po over 1h, then 1.25g po Q 1h for 8h.	C
Aminophylline	*Liquid:* 105mg/ml *Tab:* 100, 200mg *Tab (LA):* 225mg *Supp:* 250, 500mg *Inj:* 25 or 50mg/ml	***Bronchospasm:*** **PO:** *Child 1-9y.o.:* 6.7mg/kg Q 6h. *Child 9-12y.o.:* 5mg/kg Q 6h. *Child 12-16y.o.:* 4mg/kg Q 6h. *Child 16y.o.-adult:* 3.13mg/kg Q 6h. **IV load:** *Child/adult:* 6mg/kg lean body weight over 20min. **IV maintenance:** *Neonates:* 0.2mg/kg/h. *6wk-6mo.:* 0.5mg/kg/h. *6mo.-1y.o.:* 0.6-0.7mg/kg/h. *1-9y.o.:* 1.0-1.2mg/kg/h. *9-12y.o. and young adult smokers:* 0.9mg/kg/h. *Adult non-smokers:* 0.5mg/kg/h. *Adult smokers:* 0.8mg/kg/h. *Adult, older or with cor pulmonale:* 0.3mg/kg/h. *Adult with CHF/liver disease:* 0.1-0.2mg/kg/h.	C

Medication	Preparation	Dosing	Pregnancy Risk
Amiodarone (Cordarone)	Tab: 200, 400mg Inj: 50mg/ml Liquid: 50mg/ml	PO: Adult: 800-1600mg QD for 1-3wk, then 600-800mg QD for 4wk, then 200-400mg QD. Divide doses for side effects. IV: Stable: Adult: 150mg over 10min. Cardiac arrest with ventricular arrhythmia: 300mg, may repeat 150mg prn. Infusion: 1mg/min for 6h, then 0.5mg/min.	D
Amitriptyline (Elavil, Endep)	Tab: 10, 25, 50, 75, 100, 150mg Inj: 10mg/ml	Child 12-18y.o.: 25-100mg/d divided BID-TID Adult: 50-300mg po QD or 20-30mg IV Q 6h. Elderly adult: 25-150mg hs.	C
Amlodipine (Norvasc)	Tab: 2.5, 5, 10mg	Adult: HTN: 2.5-10mg QD. Angina: 5-10mg QD.	C
Amlodipine/ atorvastatin (Caduet)	Tab: 5/10, 5/20, 5/40, 5/80, 10/10, 10/20, 10/40, 10/80mg	Adult: 1 tab QD. Max: amlodipine 10mg, atorvastatin 80mg.	X
Amoxapine (Asendin)	Tab: 25, 50, 100, 150mg	Maintenance: Adult: 100-300mg/d divided BID-TID.	C

See index for proprietary names of generic meds

Amoxicillin *(Amox, Amoxil, Polymox, Trimox, Wymox)*	*Liquid:* 125, 250, 400mg/5ml *Tab:* 500, 875mg *Tab (chew):* 125, 250mg *Cap:* 250, 500mg	*Child:* 8-17mg/kg Q 8h. *Otitis media when resistant S. pneumoniae suspected:* 25-30mg/kg TID. *Adult:* 250-500mg Q 8h. *Severe disease:* 875mg po BID.	B
Amoxicillin/ clavulanate *(Augmentin)*	*Liquid:* All per 5ml: A 125mg/C 31.25mg; A 200mg/C 28.5mg; A 250mg/C 62.5mg; A 400mg/C 57mg; A 600mg/C 42.9mg; A 250mg/C 62.5mg *Tab (chew):* A 125mg/C 31.25mg; A 200mg/C 28.5mg; A 250mg/C 62.5mg; A 400mg/C 57mg *Tab:* A 250mg/C 125mg; A 500mg/C 125mg; A 875mg/C 125mg *Tab (ER):* 1000/62.5mg	*Child <3mo.:* as amoxicillin, 15mg/kg po BID. *Child >3mo., <40kg:* as amoxicillin, 13-22mg/kg po BID. *Otitis media when resistant S. pneumoniae suspected:* as amoxicillin, 40-45mg/kg po BID. *Child>40kg-adult:* as amoxicillin, 250-500mg Q 8h or 875-1000mg po BID.	B

Medication	Preparation	Dosing	Pregnancy Risk
Ampicillin *(Omnipen, Polycillin, Principen, Totacillin)*	*Liquid:* 125, 250mg/5ml *Cap:* 250, 500mg *Inj:* 125, 250, 500, 1000, 2000mg/dose	**PO:** *Child:* 12-25mg/kg Q 6h, max 2-3g/d. *Adult:* 250-1000mg Q 6h. **IM/IV:** *Child <7d, <2kg:* 25-50mg/kg Q 12h. *Child <7d, ≥2kg:* 25-33mg/kg Q 8h. *Child 7d-1mo, <1.2kg:* 25-50mg/kg Q 12h. *Child 7d-1mo, 1.2-2kg:* 25-33mg/kg Q 8h. *Child 7d-1mo, >2kg:* 25-50mg/kg Q 6h. *Child >1mo:* **Mild-moderate infections:** 25-50mg/kg Q 6h. **Severe infections:** 33-66mg/kg Q 4h or 50-100mg/kg Q 6h. *Adult:* 0.5-3g Q 4-6h, max 14g/d.	B
Ampicillin/ sulbactam *(Unasyn)*	*Inj:* Am 1g/Su 0.5g (1.5g) Am 2g/Su 1g (3.0g)	*Child >12y,o.,adult:* 1.5-3g IM/IV Q 6h.	B
Amprenavir *(Agenerase)*	*Liquid:* 15mg/ml *Cap:* 50, 150mg	*Child >13y,o.,adult:* 1200mg BID.	C
Amrinone *(Inocor)*	*Inj:* 5mg/ml	*Adult:* 0.75mg/kg IV over 2min, then 5-10µg/kg/min infusion, max 18mg/kg/d.	C
Anistreplase *(Eminase)*	*Inj:* 30U/vial	*Acute MI:* *Adult:* 30U IV over 2-5min.	C
Antipyrine/ benzocaine *(Auralgan)*	*Otic sltn:* Antipyrine 5.4%, Benzo 1.4%	*Acute OM:* *Child/adult:* fill external ear canal Q 1-2h prn. *Cerumen impaction:* fill canal TID for 2-3d before cerumen removal.	C

See index for proprietary names of generic meds

Aripiprazole (*Abilify*)	*Tab:* 5, 10, 15, 20, 30mg	*Adult:* 10-15mg QD; max 30 mg/d.	C
Aspirin	*Tab:* 81mg (*chew*), 162, 325, 500, 650, 975mg *Supp:* 120, 125, 200, 300, 325, 600, 650mg	*Child:* 10-15mg/kg po Q 4h, max 4g/d. *Adult:* varies with disease.	C,D3
Atazanavir (*Reyataz*)	*Cap:* 100, 150, 200mg	*Adult:* 400mg QD, with efavirenz/ritonavir 300mg QD.	B
Atenolol (*Tenormin*)	*Tab:* 25, 50, 100mg *Inj:* 5mg/10ml	***HTN/angina:*** *Adult:* 50-100mg po QD. ***Acute MI:*** 5mg IV over 5-10min, then 5mg IV 10min later. Give 50mg po 10min after IV dosing completed, then 50mg po in 12h.	D
Atorvastatin (*Lipitor*)	*Tab:* 10, 20, 40, 80mg	*Adult:* Start at 10mg QD, titrate Q 2wk, max 80mg/d.	X
Atovaquone (*Mepron*)	*Liquid:* 750mg/5ml *Tab:* 250mg	***PCP treatment:*** *Adult:* 750mg BID with high-fat meals for 21d. ***PCP prophylaxis:*** *Adult:* 1500mg po QD.	C

Medication	Preparation	Dosing	Pregnancy Risk
Atracurium (*Tracrium*)	*Inj:* 10mg/ml	***Initial:*** *Child 1mo.-2y.o.:* 0.3-0.4mg/kg IV push. *Child >2y.o.-adult:* 0.4-0.5mg/kg IV push. After 20-45min may repeat with 0.08-0.1mg/kg, then 0.08-0.1mg/kg Q 15-25min. ***Maintenance of paralysis:*** *Child/adult:* only after evidence of recovery from initial dose, give 9-10μg/kg/min until spontaneous recovery halted, then 5-13μg/kg/min to maintain paralysis.	C
Atropine	*Inj:* 0.05, 0.1, 0.3, 0.4, 0.5, 0.8, or 1.0mg/ml	***Heart block:*** *Child:* 0.01-0.02mg/kg/dose IV/ET. *Minimum dose 0.1mg, max 1.0mg. Adult:* 0.5-1.0mg IV/ET Q 5min. Max total 3mg. ***Asystole:*** *Child:* 0.02mg/kg/dose IV/ET Q 5min for 2-3 doses. *Adult:* 1.0mg initially, repeat Q 3-5min prn. ***Reversal of non-depolarizing paralyzing agents:*** *Child:* 0.03mg/kg 30sec before neostigmine. *Adult:* 0.5mg 30sec before neostigmine.	C

See index for proprietary names of generic meds

Atropine ophthalmic	*Sltn:* 0.5%, 1, 2% in 2ml and 5ml	***Uveitis:*** *Child:* 1-2 drops of 0.5% up to TID. *Adult:* 1-2 drops of 1% or 2% up to QID.	C
Azathioprine (Imuran)	*Cap:* 50mg *Inj:* 100mg pwd	***Renal transplant:*** *Adult:* 1-5mg/kg QD. ***Rheumatoid arthritis:*** *Adult:* 1-2.5mg/kg QD-BID.	D
Azelastine (Astelin)	*Nasal spray:* 137μg/spray	***Seasonal allergic rhinitis:*** *Child >12y.o.-adult:* 2 sprays per nostril BID.	C
Azithromycin (Zithromax)	*Oral powder:* 100, 200, 1000mg *Cap:* 250mg *Tab:* 250, 600mg *Inj:* 500mg	*Child >6mo.-16y.o.:* ***Pneumonia:*** 10mg/kg po/IV (max 500mg) once day 1, then 5mg/kg (max 250mg) po QD days 2-5. ***Otitis media:*** 30mg/kg po single dose or 10mg/kg po once, followed by either 10mg/kg po QD for 2d or 5mg/kg for 4d. *Child >16y.o.-adult:* 500mg po/IV once on day 1, then 250mg po/IV QD days 2-5. ***GC ure-thritis:*** 1g po single dose. ***Chancroid/NGU:*** 1g po. ***MAC prevention:*** 1200mg po Q wk.	B
Aztreonam (Azactam)	*Inj:* 0.5, 1, 2g	*Child >1mo.:* 30mg/kg (max 2g) IV Q 6-8h. *Adult:* 1-2g IV/IM Q 6-8h.	B
Bacitracin ophthalmic	*Cream:* 500 U/g in 3.5g	*Adult:* Apply to conjunctival sac Q 3-4h. ***Blepharitis:*** Remove crust, then apply evenly over lid margins.	C

(continued on following page)

(continued)

Medication	Preparation	Dosing	Pregnancy Risk
Bacitracin/ neomycin/ polymyxin B ophthalmic *(AKSpore, Ocutricin)*	*Cream:* 3.5g tube with (P: 10,000U/ N: 3.5mg/B: 400U) per g	*Adult:* Apply Q 3-4h for 7-10d.	D
Baclofen *(Lioresal)*	*Tab:* 10, 20mg	*Child >2y.o.:* start 5mg/kg TID. *Max 2-7y.o.: 40mg/d; max >7y.o.: 60 mg/d.* *Adult:* start 5mg TID, increase by 5mg TID Q 3d until desired effect attained. Max dose 20mg TID-QID.	C
Beclomethasone *(Vanceril, Beclovent, Beconase, Beconase AQ, Vancenase AQ)*	*Inhaler:* 42μg/puff *Nasal spray:* 42μg/spray	**Inhaler:** *Child 6-12y.o.:* 1-2 puffs Q 6-8h, max 10 puffs/d. *Child >12y.o.-adult:* 2-4 puffs Q 6-8h, max 20 puffs/d. **Nasal spray:** *Child 6-12y.o.:* 1 spray each nostril TID-QID. *Child 12y.o.-adult:* 2 sprays each nostril BID-QID.	C
Benazepril *(Lotensin)*	*Tab:* 5, 10, 20, 40mg	*Adult:* 10-40mg/d QD or divided BID. **CHF:** 5-10mg po QD.	C,D2-3
Benztropine mesylate *(Cogentin)*	*Tab:* 0.5, 1, 2mg *Inj:* 1 mg/ml	**Dystonic reaction:** *Adult:* 1-2mg IV/IM, then 1-2mg po BID for 3d.	C
Bepridil *(Vascor)*	*Tab:* 200, 300mg	*Adult:* 200-400mg QD.	C

See index for proprietary names of generic meds

			C,D2-3
Betaxolol (*Kerlone*)	*Tab:* 10, 20mg	*Adult:* 10-40mg QD.	
Betaxolol ophthalmic (*Betoptic, Betoptic S*)	*Sltn:* 0.5% in 5, 10, 15ml *Susp:* 0.25% in 2.5, 10, 15ml	*Glaucoma: Adult:* 1-2 drops in affected eye BID.	C
Bethanechol (*Urecholine, Duvoid*)	*Tab:* 5, 10, 25, 50mg *Inj:* 5mg/ml	**PO:** *Adult:* 10-50mg BID-QID. **SC:** *Adult:* 2.5mg Q 15min prn up to 4 doses, then give sum of initial doses Q 6h. *Never give IV or IM.*	C
Bicarbonate, sodium	*Tab:* 325mg, 1g *Inj:* 44, 50mEq/50ml; 5, 10mEq/10ml; 2.5mEq/5ml	**CPR:** *Child/adult:* 1mEq/kg IV Q 10min. *[Use solution of 0.5mEq/ml for child <2y.o., 1mEq/ml for others.]* **Metabolic acidosis:** *Adult:* 325mg-2g po QID.	C
Bimatoprost (*Lumigan*)	*Sltn:* 0.03%	*Adult:* 1 drop in affected eye qpm.	C
Biperiden (*Akineton*)	*Tab:* 2mg *Inj:* 5mg/ml	***Parkinson's:*** 2mg TID-QID, max 16 mg/d. **Extra-pyramidal syndrome:** 2mg QD-TID or 2mg Q 30min IM/IV to max 8mg.	C
Bisacodyl (*Dulcolax*)	*Tab:* 5mg *Supp:* 10mg	**PO:** *Child <12y.o.:* 5-10mg QD. *Child >12y.o.-adult:* 5-15mg QD. **PR:** *Child <2y.o.:* 5mg QD. *Child 2-11y.o.:* 5-10mg QD. *Child >11y.o.-adult:* 10mg QD.	B

Medication	Preparation	Dosing	Pregnancy Risk
Bisoprolol fumarate *(Zebeta)*	*Tab:* 5, 10mg	*Adult:* 5-40mg QD.	C,D2-3
Bitolterol *(Tornalate)*	*Inhaler:* 370µg/puff *Inhalation sltn:* 0.2%	**Inhaler:** *Child >12y.o.-adult:* 2-3 puffs Q 6-8h. **Nebulizer:** *Child >12y.o.-adult:* 0.5-1ml (1-2mg) TID-QID.	C
Bretylium *(Bretylol)*	*Inj:* 50mg/ml	**IV:** *Child >12y.o.-adult:* initial dose 5mg/kg/dose, then 10mg/kg/dose Q 15-30min; max total 30mg/kg. **IV infusion:** 1-2mg/min.	C
Brimonidine ophthalmic *(Alphagan)*	*Sltn:* 0.2% in 5ml and 10ml	*Glaucoma: Adult:* 1 drop in affected eye Q 8h.	B
Brinzolamide ophthalmic *(Azopt)*	*Susp:* 1% in 2.5, 5, 10, and 15ml	*Glaucoma: Adult:* 1 drop in affected eye TID.	C
Bromocriptine *(Parlodel)*	*Tab:* 2.5mg *Cap:* 5mg, 10mg	*Parkinson's:* 1.25mg BID-30mg TID. *Hyperprolactinemia:* 2.5mg BID-TID. *Acromegaly:* 1.25-30mg/d div QD-TID. *Prolactin adenomes:* 1.25-10mg/d div QD or BID.	C
Budesonide *(Rhinocort)*	*Nasal spray:* 32µg/spray	*Seasonal/perennial allergic rhinitis: Child >6y.o.-adult:* 2 sprays each nostril BID or 4 sprays each nostril QD.	C

See index for proprietary names of generic meds

			C,D(Htn)
Bumetanide *(Bumex)*	*Tab:* 0.5, 1, 2mg *Inj:* 0.25mg/ml	**PO:** *Child >1mo.:* 0.015-0.1mg/kg QD or BID. *Adult:* 0.5-2mg QD or BID, max 10mg/d. **IM/IV:** *Child >1mo.:* 0.015-0.1mg/kg/dose. *Adult:* 0.5-1.0mg over 1-2min. *For both child and adult, may repeat in 2h, max 10mg/d.*	
Bupropion *(Wellbutrin, Zyban)*	*Tab:* 75, 100mg *Tab SR:* 100, 150mg *Tab EX:* 300mg	**Antidepressant:** *Adult:* 100mg BID, increase Q 3d (max 150mg TID). Tab SR: 150mg QD-200mg BID. Tab EX: 150mg for 3d, then increase to 300mg QD. **Smoking cesssation:** *Adult:* 150mg SR QD for 3d, then increase to BID for 7-12wk.	B
Buspirone *(BuSpar)*	*Tab:* 5, 10, 15mg	*Adult:* start 5mg TID. Dose may be increased by 5mg/d every 2-4d. Max 60 mg/d.	B
Butoconazole *(Femstat, Mycelex-3)*	*Cream:* 2%	**Vaginal candidiasis:** 1 full applicator hs for 3-6d.	C
Butorphanol *(Stadol)*	*Inj:* 1 or 2mg/ml *Nasal spray:* 10mg/ml	**IM:** *Adult:* 1-4mg Q 3-4h prn. **IV:** *Adult:* 0.5-2.0mg Q 3-4h prn. **Nasal spray:** *Adult:* 1-2mg (1-2 sprays) Q 3-4h prn.	D
Caffeine	*Inj:* 500mg/2ml	**Spinal headache:** 500mg IV over 1h; may repeat in 8h.	B

Medication	Preparation	Dosing	Pregnancy Risk
Calcitonin *(Calcimar, Miacalcin)*	*Inj:* 200 IU/ml *Spray:* 200 IU/spray	***Hypercalcemia:*** 4IU/kg Q 12h IM/SC. ***Paget's:*** 50-100IU QD or QOD IM/SC. ***Bone mets with intractable pain:*** 100IU/d SC. ***Postmenopausal osteoporosis:*** 200IU (1 spray) intranasally QD, alternating nostrils.	C
Calcitriol *(Rocaltrol) po form (Calcijex) IV form*	*Cap:* 0.25, 0.5μg *Inj:* 1, 2μg/ml *Liquid:* 1μg/ml	***Renal failure: PO:*** *Child:* 0.01-0.05μg/kg/d. Titrate by 0.005-0.01μg/kg/d Q 4-8wk. *Adult:* 0.25-1.0μg QD. **IV:** *Child:* 0.01-0.05 μg/kg 3 times/wk. *Adult:* 0.5-3.0μg 3 times/wk.	D
Calcium chloride	*Inj:* 100mg (1.36mEq)/ml in 10ml	***Cardiac arrest:*** *Child:* 20mg (0.2ml)/kg IV Q 10min prn. *Adult:* 250-500mg (2.5-5.0ml) IV Q 10min prn.	C
Calcium gluconate	*Inj:* 100mg (0.46mEq)/ml in 10ml	***Cardiac arrest:*** *Child:* 50-100mg (1.0ml)/kg IV Q 10min prn. *Adult:* 0.5-1.0g (5-10ml) IV Q 10min prn. *Calcium chloride generally preferred.*	C
Candesartan *(Atacand)*	*Tab:* 4, 8, 16, 32mg	*Adult:* 8-32mg/d QD or divided BID. Usual starting dose 16mg QD.	C,D2-3
Capsaicin *(Zostrix)*	*Cream:* 0.025%, 0.075%	*Child >2y.o-adult:* apply to affected area of skin TID-QID. *May take several weeks for results.*	NR

Captopril (*Capoten*)	*Tab:* 12.5, 25, 50, 100mg	*Child <1mo.:* 0.1-0.4mg/kg/d div Q 6-8h. *Child 1mo.-1y.o.:* start 0.15-0.3mg/kg, may titrate up to max dose of 6mg/kg/d div QD-QID. *Child 1-13y.o.:* 0.5-1mg/kg/d div Q 8h, may titrate to max 6mg/kg/d, div QD-QID. *Child >13y.o.:* 12.5-25mg TID, titrate by 25mg/dose Q wk to max 450mg/d. *Adult:* **HTN:** Start 25mg BID-TID. After 1-2wk may increase to 50mg BID-TID. Usual max dose 150mg/d but may titrate to max 450mg/d with diuretic. **CHF:** Start 25mg TID (use 6.25-12.5mg TID if pt may be hypovolemic). Titrate to usual max 50-100mg TID, absolute max 450mg/d. **Diabetic nephropathy:** 25mg TID. **LV dysfunction P/MI:** 3d after MI, 6.25mg on day 1, then 12.5mg TID, then up to 25mg TID over several days, then up to 50mg TID over several wk.	C,D2-3
Carbachol ophthalmic (*Carboptic, Isopto Carbachol*)	*Sltn:* 0.75%, 1.5%, 2.25%, and 3% in 15 and 30ml	**Glaucoma:** *Adult:* 2 drops in affected eye up to TID.	C

Medication	Preparation	Dosing	Pregnancy Risk
Carbamazepine *(Tegretol)*	*Liquid:* 100mg/5ml *Tab (chew):* 100, 200mg *Tab:* 200mg *Tab SR:* 100, 200, 400mg *Cap SR:* 300mg	***Seizure loading dose: PO:** Child <12y.o.:* liquid 10mg/kg. *Child >12y.o.-adult:* liquid 8mg/kg. ***Seizure maintenance: PO:** Child <6y.o.:* 10-20mg/kg/d. *Child 6-12y.o.:* 20-30mg/kg/d. *Child 12-15y.o.:* 600-1000mg/d. *Child >15y.o.:* *Adult:* 400-1200mg/d, rarely up to 1600mg/d. *Divide TID-QID. Give SR tab in same daily dose but div BID.*	D
Carbenicillin *(Geocillin)*	*Tab:* 382mg	*Child:* 7.5-12.5mg/kg QID, max 3g/d. *Adult:* 1-2 tabs Q 6h.	B
Carisoprodol *(Soma)*	*Liquid:* 350mg/ml *Tab:* 250, 350mg	*Adult:* 350mg Q 6h.	C
Carteolol *(Cartrol)*	*Tab:* 2.5, 5mg	*Adult:* **HTN:** 2.5-10mg QD. **Angina:** 2.5-60mg po QD.	C,D2-3
Carteolol ophthalmic *(Ocupress)*	*Sltn:* 1% in 5 and 10ml	**Glaucoma:** *Adult:* 1 drop in affected eye BID.	C
Carvedilol *(Coreg)*	*Tab:* 6.25, 12.5, 25mg	*Adult:* **HTN:** 6.25-25mg BID. **Angina:** 25-50mg BID. **CHF:** 3.125-50mg BID.	C,D2-3

See index for proprietary names of generic meds

Cefaclor (2ⁿᵈ-gen) *(Ceclor, Ceclor CD)*	*Liquid:* 125, 187, 250, 375mg/5ml *Cap:* 250, 500mg *SR (CD):* 375, 500mg	*Child: **Mild-moderate infection:** 7mg/kg TID. **Acute otitis media/severe infection:** 13.3mg/kg TID. Max dose 1g/d.* Adult: 250-500mg Q 8h. *SR (CD):* give Q 12h.	B
Cefadroxil (1ˢᵗ-gen) *(Duricef, Ultracef)*	*Liquid:* 125, 250, 500mg/5ml *Cap:* 500mg *Tab:* 1g	*Child:* 15mg/kg Q 12h. *Adult:* 0.5-1.0g Q 12h.	B
Cefazolin (1ˢᵗ-gen) *(Ancef, Kefzol)*	*Inj:* 0.5, 1g	*Child <7d:* 20mg/kg IM/IV Q 12h. *Child 7d-1mo., ≤2kg:* 20mg/kg IM/IV Q 12h. *Child 7d-1mo., >2kg:* 20mg/kg IM/IV Q 8h. *Child >1mo.:* 17-33mg/kg IM/IV Q 8h. *Adult:* 0.25-2g IM/IV Q 6-8h.	B
Cefdinir (3ʳᵈ-gen) *(Omnicef)*	*Liquid:* 125mg/5ml *Cap:* 300mg	*Child 6mo.-12y.o.: **OM/sinusitis/pharyngitis:** 7mg/kg Q 12h or 14mg/kg QD for 10d. **Soft tissue infection:** 7mg/kg QD for 10d. Child 12y.o.-adult: **OM/sinusitis/pharyngitis:** 300mg Q 12h or 600mg po QD for 10d. **Soft tissue infection/community-acquired pneumonia:** 300mg Q 12h for 10d.*	B

Medication	Preparation	Dosing	Pregnancy Risk
Cefditoren *(Spectracef)*	*Tab:* 200mg	*>12y.o.-adult:* ***Chronic bronchitis/CAP:*** 400mg Q 12h for 10-14d. ***Skin/soft tissue or pharyngitis:*** 200mg Q 12h × 10d. *CrCl <50ml/min* 200mg Q 12h; *CrCl <30ml/min* 200mg Q 24h. *Take with meals.*	B
Cefepime (4th-gen) *(Maxipime)*	*Inj:* 0.5, 1, 2g	*Child >2mo.:* ***Most infections:*** 50mg/kg IM/IV Q 12h. ***Meningitis/serious infection:*** 50mg/kg IM/IV Q 8h. *Max peds dose 6 g/d.* Adult: 1-2g IV Q 12h.	B
Cefixime (3rd-gen) *(Suprax)*	*Liquid:* 100mg/5ml *Tab:* 200, 400mg	*Child:* 8mg/kg (max 400mg) QD. *Adult:* 400mg QD. **GC:** see pp. 109-110.	B
Cefoperazone (3rd-gen) *(Cefobid)*	*Inj:* 1, 2g	**IM/IV:** *Child:* 100-200mg/kg/d divided Q 8-12h. *Adult:* 2-4g Q 6-12h.	B
Cefotaxime (3rd-gen) *(Claforan)*	*Inj:* 0.5, 1, 2, 10g	*Child all ages:* ***Meningitis:*** 50mg/kg IV Q 6h, max 12 g/d. *Child <7d:* **Other:** 50mg/kg IV Q 12h. *Child >7d:* **Other:** 50mg/kg IV Q 8h. *Adult:* **Meningitis:** 2g IV Q 4h. *Adult:* **Other:** 1-2g IM/IV Q 6-12h.	B

See index for proprietary names of generic meds

Cefotetan (2nd-gen) *(Cefotan)*	*Inj:* 1, 2, 10g	*Child:* 20-40mg/kg IM/IV Q 12h. *Adult:* 1-2g IM/IV Q 12h, max 6 g/d.	B
Cefoxitin (2nd-gen) *(Mefoxin)*	*Inj:* 1, 2g	*Child >3mo.:* 27-50mg/kg IM/IV Q 8h. *Adult:* 1-2g IM/IV Q 6-8h.	B
Cefpodoxime (3rd-gen) *(Vantin)*	*Liquid:* 50, 100mg/5ml *Tab:* 100, 200mg	*Child >2mo.: **Pharyngitis/otitis media/sinusitis:*** 5mg/kg Q 12h for 5d. *Adult: **UTI:*** 100mg Q 12h for 7d. ***Other:*** 200-400mg Q 12h for 7-14d.	B
Cefprozil (2nd-gen) *(Cefzil)*	*Liquid:* 125 or 250mg/ml *Tab:* 250, 500mg	*Child >6mo.:* 7.5-15mg/kg BID. ***Pharyngitis:*** 7.5 mg/kg BID. ***OM:*** 15mg/kg BID. *Adult:* 250-500mg BID.	B
Ceftazidime (3rd-gen) *(Fortaz, Tazicef, Tazidime)*	*Inj:* 0.5, 1, 2, 6, 10g	*Child <1mo.:* 30mg/kg IV Q 12h. *Child >1mo.:* 30-50mg/kg IV Q 8h, max 6 g/d. *Adult: **Meningitis:*** 2-3g IV Q 8h. *Adult: **Other:*** 1-2g IM/IV Q 8-12h.	B
Ceftibuten (3rd-gen) *(Cedax)*	*Susp:* 90, 180mg/5ml *Cap:* 400mg	*Child:* 9mg/kg QD max 400 mg/d. *Adult:* 400mg QD.	B
Ceftizoxime (3rd-gen) *(Cefizox)*	*Inj:* 0.5, 1, 2g	*Child:* 50-67mg/kg IV Q 8h, max 12 g/d. *Adult:* 1-4g IM/IV Q 8-12h.	B

Medication	Preparation	Dosing	Pregnancy Risk
Ceftriaxone (3rd-gen) *(Rocephin)*	*Inj:* 0.25, 0.5, 1.0, 2.0, 10g	*Child:* **Meningitis:** initial dose 100mg/kg IV, then 50mg/kg IV Q 12h, max 4 g/d. *Child:* **Other:** 50-75mg/kg IM/IV Q 24h. *Adult:* **Meningitis:** 2g IV Q 12h. *Adult:* **Other:** 1-2g IM/IV Q 24h. **Epididymitis:** see p. 107. **GC:** see p. 107. **PID:** see pp. 126-127.	B
Cefuroxime (2nd-gen) *(Ceftin, Kefurox, Zinacef)*	*Liquid:* 125, 250mg/5ml *Tab:* 125, 250, 500mg *Inj:* 0.75, 1.5, 7.5g	**PO:** *Child:* **Otitis media:** 15mg/kg po BID, max 1 g/d. **Other:** 10mg/kg po BID, max 500mg/d. *Adult:* 250-500mg BID. **IM/IV:** *Child >3mo.:* **Most infections:** 50-100mg/kg/d divided Q 6-8h. **Bone/joint infections:** 50mg/kg Q 8h. *Adult:* 0.75-1.5g Q 8h. Up to 3 g/dose for severe infection.	B
Celecoxib *(Celebrex)*	*Cap:* 100, 200, 400mg	**Osteoarthritis:** *Adult:* 200mg/d either QD or divided BID. **Rheumatoid arthritis:** *Adult:* 100-200mg po BID.	C,D2-3
Cephalexin (1st-gen) *(Keflex, Keftab, Keflet)*	*Liquid:* 125, 250mg/5ml *Cap:* 250, 500mg *Tab:* 250, 500mg; 1g	*Child:* **Usual dosing:** 6-12.5mg/kg Q 6h. **Strep pharyngitis:** 12.5-25mg/kg Q 12h. **OM:** 19-25mg/kg Q 6h. *Adult:* 250-1000mg Q 6-12h.	B

See index for proprietary names of generic meds

Cephalothin (1st-gen) (*Keflin, Seffin*)	*Inj:* 1, 2g	*Child:* 13-26mg/kg IM/IV Q 4-6h. *Adult:* 0.5-2.0g IM/IV Q 4-6h.	B
Cephapirin (1st-gen) (*Cefadyl*)	*Inj:* 0.5, 1.0, 2.0g	*Child >3mo.:* 10-20 mg/kg IM/IV Q 6h, max 4 g/d. *Adult:* 0.5-2.0g IM/IV Q 4-6h.	B
Cephradine (1st-gen) (*Velosef, Anspor*)	*Liquid:* 125, 250mg/5ml *Cap:* 250, 500mg	*Child: **Usual dosing:** 6-12.5mg/kg Q 6h. **Strep pharyngitis:** 12.5-25mg Q 12h. **OM:** 25-50mg/kg/d po div Q 6-12h. *Adult:* 250-1000mg Q 6h.	B
Cetirizine (*Zyrtec*)	*Liquid:* 5mg/5ml *Tab:* 5, 10mg	*Child 2-5y.o.:* start 2-5mg QD, max 5mg/d. *Child >6y.o.-adult:* 5-10mg/d.	B
Chloral hydrate	*Liquid:* 500mg/5ml *Cap:* 250, 500mg *Supp:* 324, 500, 648mg	***Sedation for procedures:** Child:* 25-100mg/kg po/pr. ***Sleep:** Child:* 50-75mg/kg po/pr (max 1g/dose or 2 g/d). *Adult:* 500-1000mg po/pr (max 1g/dose or 2 g/d).	C
Chloramphenicol (*Chloromycetin*)	*Inj:* 1g	*Child <14d:* 6.25mg/kg Q 6h. *Child >14d- 1y.o., ≤2kg:* 12mg/kg Q 12h. *Child >14d- 1y.o., >2kg:* 25mg/kg Q 12h. *Child >1y.o.:* **Meningitis:** 25mg/kg Q 6h. *Child >1y.o.:* **Other:** 12.5-19mg/kg Q 6h, max 4 g/d. *Adult:* **Meningitis:** 12.5-25mg/kg Q 6h, max 4 g/d. *Adult:* **Other:** 12.5mg/kg Q 6h.	C

(continued on following page)

(continued)

Medication	Preparation	Dosing	Pregnancy Risk
Chloramphenicol ophthalmic *(AK-Chlor, Chloromycetin)*	*Sltn:* 5mg/ml in 7.5 and 15ml *Ointment:* 10mg/g in 3.5g	*Adult:* 2 drops of solution or a small ribbon of ointment in affected eye Q 3h for 48h, then can decrease frequency.	C
Chlordiazepoxide *(Librium)*	*Cap/tab:* 5, 10, 25mg *Inj:* 100mg/vial	**PO:** *Child >6y.o.:* 5-10mg BID-TID. *Adult:* 5-25mg TID-QID. **IM/IV:** *Adult:* 50-100mg/dose prn.	D
Chlordiazepoxide/clidinium *(Librax)*	*Cap:* Chlor 5mg/Clid 2.5mg	*Adult:* 1-2 tabs po before meals and hs.	D
Chlorhexidine *(Peridex)*	*Rinse:* 0.12% sltn	*Gingivitis: Child/adult:* 0.5oz mouth rinse for 30sec BID.	B
Chloroquine *(Aralen)*	*Tab:* 250mg of salt (=150mg of base), 500mg of salt (=300mg of base) *Inj:* 50mg of salt/ml (=40mg of base)	*All doses given as base.* *Malaria treatment:* **PO:** *Child:* 10mg/kg (max 600mg), then in 6h 5 mg/kg (max 300mg), then 5mg/kg QD (max 300mg) for 2d. *Adult:* 600mg, then in 6h 300mg, then 300mg QD for 2d. **IM:** *Child:* 5mg/kg, repeat in 6h, max 10mg/d. *Adult:* 160-200mg, repeat in 6h. Complete Rx with po doses over 2d as described previously; *Malaria prophylaxis:* **PO:** *Child:* 5mg/kg (max 300mg) Q wk. *Adult:* 300mg Q wk. Start 1-2wk before exposure, continue to 4wk after travel.	C

Chlorothiazide *(Diuril)*	*Liquid:* 250mg/5ml *Tab:* 250, 500mg *Inj:* 500mg/vial	*Child <6mo.:* 10-20mg/kg po/IV Q 12h. *Child >6mo.:* 10mg/kg po/IV Q 12h. *Adult:* 0.5-2g/d po/IV divided Q 12-24h.	C,D(Htn)
Chlorpheniramine *(Chlor-Trimeton)*	*Liquid:* 2mg/5ml *Tab:* 4mg *SR cap or tab:* 8, 12mg *Inj:* 10mg/ml, 100mg/ml	**PO:** *Child 2-6y.o.:* 1mg Q 4-6h. *Child 6-12y.o.:* 2mg Q 4-6h. *Child >12y.o.-adult:* 4mg Q 4-6h. <u>SR cap/tab:</u> 8-12mg Q 12h. **SC/IM/IV:** *Adult:* 40mg, max dose 40mg/d.	B
Chlorpromazine *(Thorazine)*	*Liquid:* 30 or 100mg/ ml; 10mg/5ml *Tab:* 10, 25, 50, 100, 200mg *SR Cap:* 30, 75, 150mg *Supp:* 25, 100mg *Inj:* 25mg/ml	***Nausea/vomiting:* PO:** *Child:* 0.5-1mg/kg Q 4-6h. *Adult:* 10-25mg Q 4-6h. **PR:** *Child >6mo.:* 1mg/kg Q 6-8h. *Adult:* 50-100mg Q 6-8h. **IM:** *Child >6mo.:* 0.5mg/kg Q 6-8h. Max <5y.o.: 40mg/d; max 5-12y.o.: 75mg/d. Adult: 10-25mg Q 4-6h.* ***Agitation in psychotic patients:* IM:** *Child >6mo.:* 0.5-1mg/kg/dose. *Adult:* initial dose 25mg, may repeat 25-50mg in 1h prn. **PO:** *Child >6mo.:* 0.5mg/kg Q 4-6h. Max <5y.o.: 40mg/d, max 5-12y.o.: 75 mg/d. Adult: 30-400mg/d divided BID-QID.*	C
Chlorpropamide *(Diabinese)*	*Tab:* 100, 250mg	*Adult:* 100-750mg po QD.	C
Chlorthalidone *(Hygroton)*	*Tab:* 15, 25, 50, 100mg	*Child:* 0.3mg/kg QD, max 50mg/d. *Adult:* 15-20mg QD.	B,D(Htn)

Medication	Preparation	Dosing	Pregnancy Risk
Chlorzoxazone *(Parafon Forte)*	*Tab:* 250, 500mg	*Child:* 5mg/kg Q 6-8h. *Adult:* 250-750mg Q 6-8h.	C
Cholestyramine *(Questran)*	*Powder:* 5g and 9g packs, each contains 4g of drug	*Child:* 240mg/kg/d divided TID. *Dose in g of drug.* *Adult:* 4g (1 pack) 1-6 times/d. *Dose in g of drug.*	B
Cidofovir *(Vistide)*	*Inj:* 75mg/ml	***CMV retinitis with AIDS:*** *Adult:* 5mg/kg IV Q wk for 2 doses, then 5mg/kg every 2wk. *Must give probenecid 2g po 3h before each dose, then 1g po 2h and 8h after infusion is completed.*	C
Cilostazol *(Pletal)*	*Tab:* 50, 100mg	*Adult:* 50-100mg BID.	C
Cimetidine *(Tagamet)*	*Liquid:* 300mg/5ml *Tab:* 100 (OTC), 200, 300, 400, 800mg *Inj:* 150mg/ml	*Child <1y.o.:* **PO/IM/IV:** 2.5-5.0mg/kg Q 6h. *Child >1y.o.:* **PO/IM/IV:** 5-10mg/kg Q 6h. *Adult:* **Active gastric/duodenal ulcer: PO:** 800mg hs, or 400mg BID, or 300mg QID. **IM/IV:** 300mg Q 6-8h. **Maintenance duodenal ulcer:** 400mg po hs. **Prevention of UGI bleed:** 50mg/h continuous infusion. **GERD:** 800mg po BID or 400mg po QID.	B
Cinoxacin *(Cinobac)*	*Cap:* 250, 500mg	**UTI:** *Adult >18y.o.:* 1g/d divided BID or QID.	C

See index for proprietary names of generic meds

Ciprofloxacin *(Cipro, Cipro XR)*	*Susp:* 250, 500mg/5ml *Tab:* 250, 500, 750mg *Tab XR:* 500, 1000mg *Inj:* 200, 400mg	**PO:** *Adult >18y.o.:* 250-750mg BID. **UTI:** *Adult:* 250mg po BID. <u>Tab XR:</u> 500mg po QD. **IV:** *Adult >18y.o.:* 200-400mg Q 8-12h. *400mg IV = 750mg po.*	C
Ciprofloxacin ophthalmic *(Ciloxan)*	*Sltn:* 3.5mg/ml in 2.5 and 5ml	*Adult:* 1-2 drops Q 2h while awake for 2d, then 1-2 drops Q 4h for the next 5d.	C
Cisatracurium *(Nimbex)*	*Inj:* 2 or 10mg/ml	**Paralysis for intubation:** *Child 2-12y.o.:* 0.1mg/kg IV, infusion 1-3µg/kg/min, titrate. *Adult:* 0.15-0.2mg/kg IV, infusion 1-3µg/kg/min, titrate.	B
Citalopram *(Celexa)*	*Tab:* 20, 40mg	**Depression:** *Adult:* 20-40mg QD.	C
Clarithromycin *(Biaxin, Biaxin XL)*	*Tab:* 250, 500mg *Tab XL:* 500mg *Susp:* 125, 250mg/5ml	**PO:** *Child:* 7.5mg/kg (max 500mg) BID. *Adult:* 250-500mg BID. <u>Tab XL:</u> 1000mg po QD.	C
Clemastine *(Tavist)*	*Syrup:* 0.67mg/5ml *Tab:* 1.34, 2.68mg	*Child 6-12y.o.:* 0.67-1.34mg BID. *Child >12y.o.-adult:* 1.34-2.68mg QD-TID.	B
Clindamycin *(Cleocin)*	*Liquid:* 75mg/5ml *Cap:* 75, 150, 300mg *Inj:* 150, 300, 600, 900mg	**PO:** *Child:* 2.0-6.3 mg/kg (max 450mg) Q 6h. *Adult:* 150-450mg Q 6h. **IM/IV:** *Child <1mo.:* 5mg/kg Q 6h. *Child >1mo.:* 5-10mg/kg Q 6-8h. *Adult:* 150-900mg Q 6h.	B

Medication	Preparation	Dosing	Pregnancy Risk
Clioquinol *(Vioform)*	*Cream, ointment:* 3%	***Eczema, tinea pedis, tinea cruris:*** Apply BID-TID daily for a maximum of 1wk.	NR
Clofazimine *(Lamprene)*	*Cap:* 50, 100mg	***MAC:*** *Adult:* 100-300mg QD with rifampin, ethambutol, ciprofloxacin.	C
Clofibrate *(AtromidS)*	*Cap:* 500mg	*Adult:* 1-2g/d in 2-4 divided doses.	C
Clonazepam *(Klonopin)*	*Tab:* 0.5, 1, 2mg	***Seizure maintenance:*** *Child <10y.o. or <30kg:* 0.003-0.01mg/kg Q 8h. *Child >10y.o. or >30kg:* 0.5mg TID. *Adult:* 0.5-6.5mg Q 8h.	D
Clonidine *(Catapres)*	*Tab:* 0.1, 0.2, 0.3mg *Patch:* TTS-1, TTS-2, TTS-3	**PO:** *Child:* 5-25μg/kg/d divided BID-QID, max 0.9mg/d. *Adult:* 0.1-1.2mg BID. **Patch:** Q wk. Patches deliver 0.1, 0.2, or 0.3mg/d.	C
Clopidogrel *(Plavix)*	*Tab:* 75mg	*Adult:* 75mg QD. ***Unstable angina going to cath lab:*** 300mg loading dose.	B
Clorazepate *(Tranxene)*	*Tab/cap:* 3.75, 7.5, 15mg *Tab SR:* 11.25, 22.5mg	***Seizure maintenance:*** *Child 9-12y.o.:* 3.75-30mg BID. *Child >12y.o.-adult:* 3.75-30mg TID. ***Anxiety:*** *Adult:* 15-60mg/d div BID-TID or (SR) 11.25-22.5mg QD.	D

See index for proprietary names of generic meds

Clotrimazole (*Lotrimin, Mycelex*)	*Tab (vag):* 100, 500mg Oral troche: 10mg Lotion, cream, sltn: 1%	***Vaginal candidiasis:*** in vagina hs for 1d (500mg) or hs for 3d (two 100mg tabs) or hs for 7d (100mg). ***Thrush/candidal esophagitis:*** *Child >3y.o.-adult:* 1 troche dissolved slowly in mouth 5 times/d for 14d. ***Tinea corporis, tinea cruris, tinea pedis, and cutaneous candidiasis:*** apply cream BID for 2-3wk.	B
Cloxacillin (*Cloxapen, Tegopen*)	*Liquid:* 125mg/5ml *Cap:* 250, 500mg	*Child >1mo.:* 12-25mg/kg (max 500mg) Q 6h. *Adult:* 250-500mg Q 6h.	B
Clozapine (*Clozaril*)	*Tab:* 25, 100mg	*Adult:* start 25mg QD-BID, increase by 25-50mg/d to 300-450mg/d, max 600-900mg/d.	B
Codeine	*Liquid:* 15mg/5ml *Tab:* 15, 30, 60mg *Inj:* 15, 30, or 60mg/ml	*Child:* 0.5-1.0mg/kg (max 60mg) po/IM/SC Q 4-6h. *Adult:* 15-60mg po/IM/SC Q 4-6h.	D
Colchicine	*Tab:* 0.5, 0.6mg *Inj:* 1mg/2ml	***Gout maintenance:*** *Adult:* 0.5-0.6mg po QOD-QD. ***Acute gout attack:*** see p. 110.	C

Medication	Preparation	Dosing	Pregnancy Risk
Colestipol (***Colestid***)	*Packet:* Granules 5g *Bulk granules:* 5 g/scoopful *Tab:* 1g	*Child:* 500mg/kg/d divided QD-QID. *Adult:* 5-30g/d divided BID-QID.	NR
Cromolyn sodium (***Intal, Nasal-Crom***)	*Inhaler:* 800μg/puff *Inhalation sltn:* 20mg/2ml *Nasal sltn:* 5.2mg per metered spray	**Asthma prevention:** *Children >5y.o.-adult:* 2 sprays from inhaler as needed up to QID. **Allergic rhinitis:** *Children >5y.o.-adult:* 1 spray in each nostril 3-6 times/d.	B
Cromolyn sodium ophthalmic (***Crolom***)	*Sltn:* 4% in 2.5 and 10ml	**Allergic conjunctivitis:** *Adult:* 1-2 drops in each eye 4-6 times/d at regular intervals.	B
Crotamiton (***Eurax***)	*Cream, lotion:* 10%	**Scabies:** see p. 133.	C
Cyclizine (***Marezine***)	*Tab:* 50mg	**PO:** *Child 6-12y.o.:* 25mg Q 6-8h, max 75mg/d. *Child >12y.o.-adult:* 50mg Q 4-6h, max 200mg/d.	B
Cyclobenzaprine (***Flexeril***)	*Tab:* 5, 10mg	*Adult:* 5-10mg TID.	B
Cyclopentolate ophthalmic (***Cyclogyl***)	*Sltn:* 0.5%, 1%, and 2% in 2, 5 and 15ml	*Child <1y.o.:* 1 drop of 0.5%. *Child >1y.o.:* 1-2 drops. *Adult:* 1-2 drops. Compress lacrimal sac after instillation.	C

See index for proprietary names of generic meds

Drug	Formulations	Indications/Dosage	
Cyclosporine (Neoral, Sandimmune)	*Liquid:* 100mg/ml *Cap:* 25, 50, 100mg	***Maintenance of organ transplant:*** *Child/adult:* 5-10mg/kg BID.	C
Cyproheptadine (Periactin)	*Liquid:* 2mg/5ml *Tab:* 4mg	*Child 2-6y.o.:* 2mg Q 8-12h. *Child 7-14y.o.:* 4mg Q 8-12h. *Child >14y.o.-adult:* 4-20 mg/d divided Q 8h.	B
Dalteparin (Fragmin)	*Inj:* 2500U/0.2ml, 5000U/0.2ml, 7500U/0.3ml, 10,000U/ml, 25,000U/ml	*Adult:* 2500-10,000U SC QD.	B
Danazol (Danocrine)	*Cap:* 50, 100, 200mg	***Hereditary angioedema:*** *Adult:* 200mg BID-TID. ***Endometriosis:*** 100-200mg BID; if severe, max 400mg BID.	X
Dantrolene (Dantrium)	*Cap:* 25, 50, 100mg *Inj:* 20mg/vial	***Malignant hyperthermia:*** see p. 116. ***Chronic spasticity:*** *Child:* 0.5mg/kg po QD, titrate to BID-QID, max 100mg po QID. *Adult:* start 25mg po QD; may increase to BID, TID, or QID; max 100mg QID.	C
Dapiprazole ophthalmic (Rev-Eyes)	*Powder for reconstitution:* 0.5% in 5ml	***To reverse mydriasis:*** *Adult:* 2 drops, then repeat in 5min.	B

Medication	Preparation	Dosing	Pregnancy Risk
Dapsone	*Tab:* 25, 100mg	***Pneumocystis suppression:*** *Child>* 1mo: 2mg/kg (max 100mg) po QD. *Adult:* 100mg po QD.	C
Daptomycin *(Cubicin)*	*Inj:* 250, 500mg	*Adult:* 4mg/kg IV Q 24h × 7-14d.	B
Deferoxamine *(Desferal)*	*Inj:* 500mg, 2g/vial	***Iron OD:*** *Child/adult:* 15mg/kg/h infusion, max 250mg/h. See p. 60.	C
Delavirdine *(Rescriptor)*	*Tab:* 100, 200mg	***HIV:*** *Child >13y.o.-adult:* 400mg TID.	C
Desipramine *(Norpramin)*	*Tab:* 10, 25, 50, 75, 100, 150mg	***Depression:*** *Child 6-12y.o.:* 1-3mg/kg/d, divide BID-TID. *Child >12y.o.:* 25-150mg QD. *Adult:* 75-300mg QD.	C
Desloratadine *(Clarinex)*	*Tab:* 5mg	*Child >12y.o.-adult:* 5mg QD.	C
Desmopressin *(DDAVP, Stimate)*	*Nasal spray:* 150µg/spray *Inj:* 4, 15µg/ml	***Hemophilia A, von Willebrand Disease:*** see p. 79.	B
Dexamethasone *(Decadron)*	*Elixir:* 0.5mg/5ml *Oral sltn:* 0.1, 1.0mg/ml *Tab:* 0.25, 0.5, 0.75, 1.0, 1.5, 2, 4, 6mg *Inj:* 4, 8, 10, 16, 20, 24mg/ml	*Dosage dependent on disease process being treated.*	C,D1

See index for proprietary names of generic meds

Dexamethasone ophthalmic *(Decadron, AK-Dex)*	*Sltn:* 0.1% in 5ml *Susp:* 0.1% in 5 and 15ml *Ointment:* 0.05% in 3.5g	*Adult:* <u>Sltn/susp:</u> 1-2 drops Q 1h during the day, Q 2h at night until response occurs, then decrease to Q 4h or less as needed. <u>Ointment:</u> Apply thin coat TID-QID until response occurs, then decrease to BID or QD as needed.	C
Dexchlor-pheniramine *(Polaramine)*	*Tab:* 2mg *Syrup:* 2mg/5ml *Repeat tab:* 4, 6mg	*Child 2-5y.o.:* 0.5mg Q 4-6h. *Child 6-11y.o.:* 1mg Q 4-6h or 4mg repeat tab hs. *Child >12y.o.-adult:* 2mg Q 4-6h or repeat tab 4-6mg hs.	B
Diazepam *(Valium, Valrelease)*	*Liquid:* 1 or 5mg/ml *Tab:* 2, 5, 10mg *Inj:* 5mg/ml	**PO:** *Child >1mo.:* 0.03-0.2mg/kg (max 10mg) Q 6h. *Adult:* 2-10mg Q 6-12h. **IV:** *Child >1mo.:* 0.25mg/kg (max 10mg) Q 15min prn. *Adult:* 5-10mg Q 10min prn.	D
Diazoxide *(Hyperstat)*	*Inj:* 300mg/20ml	**HTN:** 1-3mg/kg IV (max 150mg) Q 5-15min, titrate until BP reaches desired level.	C
Dichlorphenamide *(Daranide)*	*Tab:* 50mg	*Adult:* **Loading dose:** 100-200mg, then 100mg Q 12h to desired response. **Maintenance:** 25-50mg QD-TID.	C
Diclofenac *(Voltaren, Voltaren XR)*	*Tab:* 25, 50, 75mg *SR:* 100mg	*Adult:* 100-200mg/d as tabs divided Q 8-12h. Use SR QD.	B,D3
Dicloxacillin *(Dynapen)*	*Liquid:* 62.5mg/5ml *Cap:* 125, 250, 500mg	*Child <40kg:* 6-12mg/kg (max 500mg) Q 6h. *Child >40kg-adult:* 125-500mg Q 6h.	B

Medication	Preparation	Dosing	Pregnancy Risk
Dicyclomine (*Bentyl*)	*Liquid:* 10mg/5ml *Cap:* 10mg *Tab:* 20mg *Inj:* 10mg/ml	*Adult:* **PO:** 20-40mg Q 6h. **IM:** 20mg IM Q 6h.	B
Didanosine (*Videx*)	*Powder for pediatric liquid:* 10mg/ml *Tab†:* 25, 50, 100, 150mg *Single-dose packets†:* 100, 167, 250, 375mg	*Tab 1mg (doses in regular type) equals 1.25mg of powder or liquid (doses in bold type).* *Child (by body surface area in m²*) <90d:* 50mg (**62mg**)/m²; *90d-13y.o.:* 90-150mg (**112-187mg**)/m². *Child 13y.o.-adult <60kg:* 125mg (**167mg**) BID. *Child >13y.o.-adult >60kg:* 200mg (**250mg**) BID.	B
	†Chew tabs thoroughly or dissolve in 1oz water. Dissolve powder in at least 1oz water. **See p. 73 for body surface area determination*		
Diflunisal (*Dolobid*)	*Tab:* 250, 500mg	*Adult:* 250-500mg Q 8-12h.	B,D3
Digoxin (*Lanoxin*)	*Liquid:* 0.05mg/ml *Tab:* 0.125, 0.25, 0.5mg *Cap:* 0.05, 0.1, 0.2mg	***Loading dose:*** *give 1/2 initially po/IM/IV, remainder in two equally divided doses Q 6-8h (po/IM) or Q 4h (IV).* ***Maintenance:*** *give indicated dose QD.*	C

See index for proprietary names of generic meds

Inj: 0.1 or 0.25mg/ml

	Loading		Maintenenance	
	PO	IM/IV	PO	IM/IV
Premature	20-30µg/kg	15-25	5-7.5µg/kg	4-6
Full term	25-35	20-30	6-10	5-8
1mo.-2y.o.	35-60	30-50	10-15	7.5-12
2-5y.o.	30-40	25-35	7.5-10	6-9
5-10y.o.	20-35	15-30	5-10	4-8
10-18y.o.	10-15	8-12	2.5-5	2-3
>10y.o.-adult	0.75-1.5mg		0.125-0.5mg	

Typical loading dose for a 70kg adult: **PO:** 0.5mg, then 0.25mg Q 6-8h for 2 doses. **IV:** 0.5mg, then 0.25mg Q 4h for 2 doses. *Both of these regimens total 3 doses and 1.0mg.*

Drug	Forms		Pregnancy
Digoxin immune Fab *(Digibind)*	*Inj:* 40mg/4ml	***Digitalis OD:*** see p. 59.	C
Dihydroergotamine mesylate *(D.H.E. 45, Migranal)*	*Nasal spray:* 0.5mg/spray *Inj:* 1mg/ml	*Adult:* **Inhaled:** 1mg spray each nostril. Repeat in 15min. **IM:** 1mg Q 1h, max 3 doses/d. **IV:** 1mg Q 1h, max 2 doses/d. Max 6mg/wk. *Consider treating for nausea before IM/IV administration.*	X
Diltiazem *(Cardizem, Cardizem LA, Cardizem XR, Dilacor XR)*	*Tab:* 30, 60, 90, 120mg *Tab (Cardizem LA):* 120, 180, 240, 300, 360, 420mg	**PO:** *Adult:* ***Angina:*** 30-90mg (tab) QID before meals and hs; or 120-480mg QD (Cardizem CD). ***HTN:*** 180-360mg QD (Cardizem CD or Dilacor XR); or 60-180mg BID (Cardizem SR); or 120-540mg QD (Cardizem LA). *(continued on following page)*	C

(continued)

Medication	Preparation	Dosing	Pregnancy Risk
Diltiazem *(continued)*	*Cap* (Cardizem SR): 60, 90, 120mg *Cap* (Cardizem CD): 120, 180, 240, 300mg *Cap* (Dilacor XR): 120, 180, 240mg *Inj:* 5mg/ml	**IV:** *Adult:* initial: 0.25mg/kg over 2min. May repeat dose of 0.35mg/kg after 15min if necessary. **Infusion:** *Adult:* start 5-10mg/h after initial IV as described previously. May increase in 5mg steps to max 15mg/h for up to 24h.	
Dimenhydrinate *(Dramamine, Dimetabs)*	*Liquid:* 12.5mg/5ml *Tab* (chew) or *cap:* 50mg *Inj:* 50mg/ml	*Child 2-6y.o.:* 1.25mg/kg po/IM Q 6h, max 75mg/d. *Child 6-12y.o.:* 1.25mg/kg po/IM Q 6h, max 150mg/d. *Adult:* 50-100mg po/IM/IV Q 4-6h, max po 400mg/d, max IM/IV 300mg/d.	B
Diphenhydramine *(Benadryl)*	*Liquid:* 12.5mg/5ml *Tab/cap:* 25, 50mg *Inj:* 10mg or 50mg/ml	**PO/IM/IV:** *Child:* 1.25mg/kg Q 6h, max 300mg/d. *Adult:* 25-50mg Q 4-6h.	B
Diphenoxylate/ atropine *(Lomotil)*	*Liquid:* Diphen 2.5mg/atropine 0.025mg per 5ml (in 15% alcohol) *Tab:* Diphen 2.5mg/atropine 0.025mg	*Child >2y.o.:* (as diphen) 0.075-0.1mg/kg QID. *Adult:* 10ml or 2 tabs QID until diarrhea is controlled.	C

See index for proprietary names of generic meds

Dipivefrin ophthalmic (*Propine, AKPro*)	*Sltn:* 0.1% in 5, 10, or 15ml	*Glaucoma: Adult:* 1 drop in affected eye Q 12h.	B
Dipyridamole (*Persantine*)	*Tab:* 25, 50, 75mg	*Adult:* 75-100mg QID.	C
Dipyridamole/aspirin (*Aggrenox*)	*Cap:* Dip 200mg/ASA 25mg	*Secondary stroke prophylaxis:* 1 cap BID.	D
Dirithromycin (*Dynabac*)	*EC Tab:* 250mg	*Child >12y.o.-adult:* 500mg QD with meals for 7-14d.	C
Disopyramide (*Norpace*)	*Cap:* 100, 150mg *Cap ER:* 100, 150mg	*Child <1y.o.:* 2.5-7.5mg/kg Q 6h. *Child 1-4y.o.:* 2.5-5.0mg/kg Q 6h. *Child 4-12y.o.:* 2.5-3.8mg/kg Q 6h. *Child 12-18y.o.:* 1.5-3.8mg/kg Q 6h. *Adult <50kg:* start 100mg Q 6h or (*Cap ER*) 200mg Q 12h. *Adult >50kg:* start 150mg Q 6h or (*Cap ER*) 300mg Q 12h. *Max adult dose may be titrated to 1600mg/d.*	C
Disulfiram (*Antabuse*)	*Tab:* 250, 500mg	*Adult:* 125-500mg QD.	C
Divalproex (*Depakote*)	*Sprinkle cap:* 125mg *Tab:* 125, 250, 500mg *Tab ER:* 500mg	*Seizures: Child 10y.o.-adult:* 10-60mg/kg/d. Divide if dose exceeds 250mg/d. *Mania: Adult:* start 375mg BID, max 60mg/kg/d. *Migraine HA: Adult:* 250-500mg BID; *Tab ER:* 500-1000mg/d.	D

Medication	Preparation	Dosing	Pregnancy Risk
Dobutamine (*Dobutrex*)	*Inj:* 250, 500, 1000, 1250mg	*Child/adult:* start 2-15μg/kg/min, max 40μg/kg/min.	B
Docusate sodium (*Colace*)	*Syrup:* 20mg/5ml *Sltn:* 10 and 50mg/ml *Tab:* 100mg *Cap:* 50, 100, 240, 250mg	*Child <3y.o.:* 10mg QD-QID. *Child 3-6y.o.:* 20mg QD-QID. *Child 6-12y.o.:* 40mg QD-QID. *Child >12y.o.-adult:* 50-125mg QD-QID.	C
Dofetilide (*Tikosyn*)	*Cap:* 125, 250, 500μg	*Afib/flutter:* 500μg BID with QTc monitoring 2h after dose. Halve dosage if QTc >15% over baseline or >500msec. Should be initiated during a 72h period of in-hospital ECG monitoring.	C
Dolasetron (*Anzemet*)	*Tab:* 50, 100mg *Inj:* 20mg/ml	**PO:** *Pre-op surgical N/V: Child 2-16y.o.:* 1.2mg/kg (max 100mg). *Child 16y.o.-adult:* 100mg. For all: give 2h before surgery. **ChemoRx N/V:** *Child 2-16y.o.:* 1.8mg/kg (max 100mg). *Child 16y.o.-adult:* 100mg. For all: give within 1h of chemoRx. **IV:** *Pre-op surgical N/V: Child 2-16y.o.:* 0.35mg/kg (max 12.5mg). *Child 16y.o.-adult:* 12.5mg. For all: give 30min before surgery ends or at onset N/V. **ChemoRx N/V:** *Child/adult:* 1.8mg/kg (max 100mg). Give 30min before chemoRx.	B

See index for proprietary names of generic meds

Donepezil *(Aricept)*	*Tab*: 5, 10mg	***Alzheimer's:*** *Adult*: 5-10mg QD.	C
Dopamine *(Intropin)*	*Inj*: 40, 80, or 160mg/ml	*Child/adult*: 2-5μg/kg/min IV = renal dose. 5-15μg/kg/min IV = renal, inotropic, and chronotropic effects. >15μg/kg/min IV = α-adrenergic effects pre- dominate.	C
Dorzolamide ophthalmic *(Trusopt)*	*Sltn*: 2% in 5 and 10ml	***IOP:*** *Adult*: 1 drop in affected eye TID.	C
Doxacurium chloride *(Nuromax)*	*Inj*: 1mg/ml	***RSI:*** *Child* >2y.o.: 0.03mg/kg IV. *Adult*: 0.05mg/kg IV. ***To maintain paralysis after initial dose:*** *Child* >2y.o.-*adult*: 0.005-0.01mg/kg prn.	C
Doxazosin *(Cardura)*	*Tab*: 1, 2, 4, 8mg	*Adult*: ***HTN:*** 1-16mg QD. ***BPH:*** 1-8mg QD.	C
Doxepin *(Sinequan)*	*Liquid*: 10mg/ml *Cap*: 10, 25, 50, 75, 100, 150mg	*Adult*: 75-300mg/d in single or divided doses.	C

Medication	Preparation	Dosing	Pregnancy Risk
Doxycycline (*Vibramycin, Doxy Caps, Doxychel Hyclate*)	*Liquid:* 25, 50mg/5ml *Tab/cap:* 50, 100mg *Inj:* 100, 200mg	**PO:** *Child >8y.o. and <45kg:* 1.1-2.2mg/kg BID. *Child >45kg-adult:* 100mg BID. **IV:** *Child >8y.o. and <45kg:* 4.4mg/kg/d on day 1 divided Q 12h, then 2.2-4.4mg/kg/d given QD or divided Q 12h, max 200mg/d. *Child >45kg-adult:* 200mg/d on day 1, given QD or divided Q 12h, then 100-200mg/d given QD or divided Q 12h.	D
Doxylamine (*Unisom*)	*Tab:* 25mg	*Adult:* 25mg hs prn.	A
Droperidol (*Inapsine*)	*Inj:* 2.5mg/ml	*Child 2-12y.o.:* 0.05-0.06mg/kg IM/IV Q 4-6h. *Adult:* 2.5-5mg IM/IV Q 3-4h. *May cause QTc prolongation and cardiac AR. Use w/caution in pts w/heart disease, possible electrolyte disorder, or on drugs which cause increased QTc.*	C
Drotrecogin alfa (*Xigris*)	*Inj:* 5, 20mg powder	*Adult:* 24µg/kg/h × 96h.	C
Dutasteride (*Avodant*)	*Cap:* 0.5mg	**BPH:** *Adult:* 0.5mg QD.	X
Ecothiophate Iodide ophthalmic (*Phospholine Iodide*)	*Powder for reconstitution:* 0.03%, 0.06%, 0.125%, and 0.25% in 5ml	*Glaucoma: Adult:* 1 drop in affected eye BID.	C

See index for proprietary names of generic meds

Edrophonium (Tensilon)	Inj: 10mg/ml	Tensilon test: IV: see page xxx.	C
Efavirenz (Sustiva)	Cap: 50, 100, 200mg Tab: 600mg	Child 10-15kg: 200mg QD. Child 15-20kg: 250mg QD. Child 20-25kg: 300mg QD. Child 25-32.5kg: 350mg QD. Child 32.5-39kg: 400mg QD. Child >39kg-adult: 600mg QD.	C
Eflornithine (Ornidyl)	Inj: 200mg/ml	Pneumocystis pneumonia: Adult: 100mg/kg IV Q 6h over 45min for 14d.	C
Eletriptan (Relpax)	Tab: 20, 40mg	Adult: 20-40mg; may repeat in 2h; max single dose 40mg, max 80mg/d.	C
Emedastine ophthalmic (Emadine)	Sltn: 0.05% in 5ml	Adult: 1 drop in affected eye up to QID.	B
Emtricitabine (Emtriva)	Cap: 200mg	Adult: 200mg QD. CrCl 30-49ml/min: 200mg Q 48h; CrCl 15-29ml/min: 200mg Q 72h; CrCl <15 and HD: 200mg Q 96h.	B
Enalapril (Vasotec)	Tab: 2.5, 5, 10, 20mg Inj: 1.25mg/ml	PO: Child: start 0.1mg/kg/d, titrate to max 0.5mg/kg/d QD or divided BID. Adult: 5-40mg/d QD or divided BID. IV: Child: 5-10µg/kg up to 3 times/d. Adult: 1.25mg Q 6h. Administer over 5min.	C,D3

Medication	Preparation	Dosing	Pregnancy Risk
Enoxaparin (*Lovenox*)	*Inj:* 30mg/0.3ml; 40mg/0.4ml; 60mg/0.6ml; 80mg/0.8ml; 100mg/ml; 120mg/0.8ml; 150mg/ml	***Acute DVT/PE:*** *Child/adult:* 1mg/kg SC Q 12h. ***Unstable angina:*** *Adult:* 1mg/kg SC Q 12h. ***DVT prophylaxis post-op knee/hip replacement:*** *Adult:* 30mg SC Q 12h for 7-14d or 40mg SC QD for 21d. ***Post-op abdominal surgery:*** 40mg SC QD for 7-12d.	B
Epinastine (*Elestat*)	*Sltn:* 0.05%	*Adult:* 1 drop in each eye BID.	C
Epinephrine	*Inj:* 1:1000 = 1g/1000ml; 1:10,000 = 1g/10,000ml	***Cardiac arrest:*** *Child <1mo.:* 0.01-0.03mg/kg IV Q 3-5min. *Child >1mo.:* 0.01mg/kg IV initially, then 0.01mg/kg (max 1mg) IV/ET Q 3-5min. *Adult:* 1mg IV/ET Q 5min. ***Anaphylaxis:*** *Child:* 0.01mg/kg (max 0.5mg) IV over 5min. *Adult:* 0.1-0.5mg IV over 5min. ***Asthma:*** *Child:* 0.01mg/kg (max 0.3mg) SC Q 20min prn × 3. *Adult:* 0.3mg SC Q 20min prn × 3.	C
Epinephrine ophthalmic (*Glaucon, Epifrin*)	*Sltn:* 0.5%, 1%, 2% in 10 and 15ml	***Glaucoma:*** *Adult:* 1 drop in affected eye QD or BID. *Instill a miotic first.*	C

See index for proprietary names of generic meds

Epinephrine, racemic	*Sltn:* 22.5mg/ml (7.5, 15, 30ml)	*Child/adult:* 0.05ml/kg (max 0.5ml)/dose (*child*) or 0.5ml (*adult*) with 2ml NS over 15min nebulized Q 1-2h prn.	C
Eplerenone (*Inspra*)	*Tab:* 25, 50, 100mg	*Adult:* **CHF:** 25mg QD after 1 mo. may increase to 50mg QD; HTN: 50mg QD, max 50mg BID; contraindicated in *CrCl <50 ml/min.*	B
Eptifibatide (*Integrilin*)	*Inj:* 75 or 2000µg/ml	*Adult:* 180µg/kg IV bolus, then 2µg/kg/min infusion for up to 72h, max 15mg (=15,000µg)/h.	B
Ergonovine	*Tab:* 0.2mg *Inj:* 0.2mg/ml	***Postpartum/post-abortion hemorrhage:*** **IM/IV:** 0.2mg IM or IV (use IV only if uterine bleeding is severe). Repeat Q 2-4h, max 5 doses. **PO:** 0.2-0.4mg po (or SL) Q 6-12h.	NR
Ergotamine (*Ergomar, Ergostat*)	*Tab SL:* 2mg	**SL:** *Child 12-18y.o.:* 1mg Q 30min. Max 3mg/d. *Adult:* 2mg, then 1-2mg Q 30min. Max 6mg/d, 10mg/wk.	X
Ergotamine/ caffeine (*Cafergot, Wigraine*)	*Tab:* Erg 1mg/Caff 100mg *Supp:* Erg 2mg/Caff 100mg	*Adult:* 2 tabs po, then 1 tab po Q 30min; or 1 supp PR, then 2nd supp 1h later if needed. *Max/attack:* 6 tabs or 2 supp. *Max/wk:* 10 tabs or 5 supp.	X
Ertapenem (*Invanz*)	*Inj:* 1g	*Adult:* 1g IV/IM QD. *CrCl 30 ml/min or HD:* 500mg IV/IM QD.	B

Medication	Preparation	Dosing	Pregnancy Risk
Erythromycin base (*E-mycin, ERYC, Ethril, Erythrocin, Robimycin*)	*Tab:* 250, 333, 500mg *Tab (enteric coated):* 250, 333, 500mg *Pellets (enteric coated):* 250mg	*Child <7d:* 10mg/kg Q 12h. *Child 7d-1mo.:* 10mg/kg Q 8h. *Child >1mo.:* 7.5-12.5mg/kg (max 500mg dose) Q 6h. *Adult:* 250-500mg Q 6h or 500mg Q 12h.	B
Erythromycin estolate (*Ilosone*)	*Drops:* 100mg/ml *Susp:* 125, 250mg/5ml *Tab:* 250, 500mg *Cap:* 125, 250mg	*Child <7d:* 10mg/kg Q 12h. *Child 7d-1mo.:* 10mg/kg Q 8h. *Child >1mo.:* 7.5-12.5mg/kg (max 500mg) Q 6h. *Adult:* 250-500mg Q 6h or 500mg Q 12h. *Avoid treatment for >10d or repeated courses to reduce chance of hepatotoxicity.*	B
Erythromycin ethylsuccinate (*E.E.S.*)	*Liquid:* 200, 400mg/5ml *Granules for oral susp:* 200, 400mg/5ml *Drops:* 100mg/2.5ml *Tab:* 200, 400mg *Tab (chew):* 200mg	*Child <7d:* 10mg/kg Q 12h. *Child 7d-1mo.:* 10mg/kg Q 8h. *Child >1mo.:* 7.5-12.5mg/kg (max 500mg dose) Q 6h. *Adult:* 400-800mg Q 6h or 800mg Q 12h. *Higher doses may be needed than for other formulations. (Guideline: 200mg = 125mg of other formulations.)*	C
Erythromycin lactobionate or gluceptate	*Inj:* 0.5, 1.0g	**IV:** *Child:* 5.0-12.5mg/kg (max 1g) Q 6h. *Adult:* 3.75-5mg (max 1g) Q 6h.	B

See index for proprietary names of generic meds

Erythromycin ophthalmic *(Ilotycin)*	*Ointment:* 5% in 3.5g	*Adult:* Apply 1cm of ointment to affected eye 6 times/d.	B
Erythromycin stearate *(Erythrocin Stearate, Erypar w/o filmseal, Ethril, Wyamycin S)*	*Tab:* 250, 500mg	*Child >1mo.:* 7.5-12.5mg/kg (max 500mg/dose) Q 6h. *Adult:* 250-500mg Q 6h or 500mg Q 12h.	B
Erythromycin/ sulfisoxazole *(Pediazole)*	*Liquid:* Erythro 200mg/Sulf 600mg/5ml	*Child >2mo.:* 0.3ml/kg (max 12.5ml) Q 6h.	C
Escitalopram *(Lexapro)*	*Liquid:* 5mg/5ml *Tab:* 5, 10, 20mg	*Adult:* usual dose 10mg QD, range 5-20mg QD.	C
Esmolol *(Brevibloc)*	*Inj:* 100mg/vial; 2.5g/ampule	*Child/adult:* 500µg/kg loading dose over 1min IV, then 50µg/kg/min infusion. If no effect in 4min, repeat loading dose and increase infusion to 100µg/kg/min. May repeat loading dose in 4min and increase infusion by 50µg/kg/min 2 additional times. Max infusion rate: *child:* 1000µg/kg/min; *adult:* 300µg/kg min.	C

Medication	Preparation	Dosing	Pregnancy Risk
Esomeprazole *(Nexium)*	*Tab:* 20, 40mg	*Adult:* 20-40mg QD.	B
Estazolam *(ProSom)*	*Tab:* 1, 2mg	*Adult:* 1-2mg hs prn.	X
Estrogens, conjugated *(Premarin)*	*Tab:* 0.3, 0.45, 0.625, 0.9, 1.25, 2.5mg *Inj:* 25mg/vial	***Menopause, atrophic vaginitis, osteoporosis:*** Cycle as follows: 0.3-1.25mg po QD for 3wk, off for 1wk. ***Heavy uterine bleeding:*** 25mg IV, may repeat Q 4h prn for 4 total doses.	X
Ethacrynic acid *(Edecrin)*	*Tab:* 25, 50mg *Inj:* 50mg/vial	*IV: Adult:* 0.5-1mg/kg, max 100mg slowly. *PO: Child >1y.o.:* start 25mg QD. May titrate in 25mg increments Q 2-3d to desired effect. *Adult:* 50-200mg QD.	B,D(Htn)
Ethambutol *(Myambutol)*	*Tab:* 100, 400mg	*TB initial Rx: Child >13y.o.-adult:* 15mg/kg QD. *TB Re-Rx: Child >13y.o.-adult:* 25mg/kg QD for 60d, then 15mg/kg QD.	B
Ethionamide *(Trecator-SC)*	*Tab:* 250mg	*Adult:* 500-1000mg/d in divided doses.	C
Ethosuximide *(Zarontin)*	*Liquid:* 250mg/5ml *Cap:* 250mg	*Seizure maintenance: Child >3y.o.:* 10-15mg/kg (max 750mg) BID. *Adult:* 250-750mg BID.	C

Etodolac **(Lodine)**	*Cap:* 200, 300mg *Tab:* 400, 500mg *Tab Extended* *Release:* 400, 500, 600mg	***Pain:*** *Adult:* 200-400mg TID-QID prn. ***DJD:*** 600-1200mg/d as 200mg TID-QID, 300mg BID-QID, or 400mg BID-TID. Tab ER: 400-1000mg po. *Max 1200mg/d; if <60kg, 20mg/kg/d.*	C,D3
Etomidate **(Amidate)**	*Inj:* 2mg/ml	***Sedation for rapid sequence intubation:*** *Child >9y.o.-adult:* 0.2-0.3mg/kg IV over 15-60sec.	C
Ezetimibe **(Zetia)**	*Tab:* 10mg	*Adult:* 10mg QD.	C
Famciclovir **(Famvir)**	*Tab:* 125, 250, 500mg	***Herpes simplex:*** see pp. 114-115. ***Herpes zoster:*** see pp. 142-143.	B
Famotidine **(Pepcid)**	*Liquid:* 40mg/5ml *Tab:* 10 (OTC), 20, 40mg *Inj:* 10mg/ml	*Child:* ***PUD:*** 0.5mg/kg/d hs po/IV or div BID, max 40mg/d. ***GERD:*** 0.5mg/kg, max 40mg, po/IV BID. *Adult:* ***PO: Duodenal ulcer, acute:*** 40mg hs or 20mg BID. ***Duodenal ulcer, maintenance:*** 20mg hs. ***Gastric ulcer, acute:*** 40mg hs. ***GERD:*** 20mg BID. ***Reflux esophagitis with*** ***erosions/ulcers:*** 20-40mg BID. **IV:** 20mg Q 12h.	B
Felbamate **(Felbatol)**	*Liquid:* 600mg/5ml *Tab:* 400, 600mg	*Child 14y.o.-adult:* 1200-3600mg/d divided TID-QID.	C
Felodipine **(Plendil)**	*Tab:* 2.5, 5, 10mg	*Adult:* usual 5-10mg QD, max 20mg QD.	C
Fenofibrate **(Tricor)**	*Tab:* 48, 145mg	*Adult:* 48-145mg QD.	C

Medication	Preparation	Dosing	Pregnancy Risk
Fenoldopam *(Corlopam)*	*Inj:* 10mg/ml (1, 2, 5ml)	***Hypertensive emergency:*** *Adult:* Start infusion at 0.03-0.1µg/kg/min. No loading dose necessary. Titrate at not less than 15min intervals in 0.05-0.1µg/kg/min increments. *Max dose:* 1.6µg/kg/min.	B
Fenoprofen *(Nalfon)*	*Tab:* 600mg *Cap:* 200, 300mg	*Adult:* **Pain:** 200mg Q 4-6h prn. ***Arthritis:*** 300-600mg TID-QID, max 3.2g/d.	B,D3
Fentanyl *(Sublimaze, Duragesic, Actiq)*	*Transmucosal lozenge:* 200, 400, 600, 800, 1200, 1600µg *Inj:* 50µg/ml *Patch:* release 25, 50, 75, 100µg/h	***Conscious sedation:*** *Child 2-12y.o.:* 2-3µg/kg IV over 3min Q 30min prn. *Child >12y.o.-adult:* 50-100µg over 3min Q 30min prn. **Chronic pain:** *Adult:* 1 patch Q 72h. *Start patients who are not tolerant of opiates with 25µg/h patch.* ***Breakthrough cancer pain:*** *Adult:* 200µg transmucosal unit over 15min. May repeat in 30min, max 4 U/d.	D
Ferrous fumarate (33% elemental iron) *(Femiron, Feostat, Fumasorb, Fumerin, Hemocyte, Ircon-FA)*	*Liquid:* 100mg/5ml *Tab:* 200, 325mg *Tab (chew):* 100mg *Tab (ER):* 325mg	***Iron deficiency anemia:*** *Adult:* 200mg TID or QID. <u>ER tab</u>: 325mg BID.	C

See index for proprietary names of generic meds

Ferrous gluconate (12% elemental iron) *(Fergon, Ferralet, Simron)*	*Tab:* 240, 325mg	***Iron deficiency anemia:*** *Child >2y.o.:* 8-16mg/kg Q 8h. *Adult:* 325mg Q 8h.	A
Ferrous sulfate (20% elemental iron) *(Feosol, Fer-In-Sol, Fer-Iron, Fero-Gradumet, Ferospace, Ferralyn, Ferra-TD, Mol-Iron, Slow Fe)*	*Elixir:* 220mg/5ml *Drops:* 75mg/0.6ml *Tab:* 160, 187, 325mg	***Iron deficiency anemia:*** *Child >2y.o.:* 5-10mg/kg Q 8h. *Adult:* 300mg Q 8h.	C
Fexofenadine *(Allegra)*	*Cap:* 60mg *Tab:* 30, 60, 180mg	*Child >12y.o.-adult:* 60mg BID or 180mg QD.	C
Finasteride *(Proscar, Propecia)*	*Tab:* 1mg (Propecia), 5mg (Proscar)	***Androgenic alopecia:*** 1mg QD. ***BPH:*** 5mg QD.	X
Flavoxate *(Urispas)*	*Tab:* 100mg	*Child >12y.o.-adult:* 100-200mg Q 6-8h.	B
Flecainide *(Tambocor)*	*Tab:* 50, 100, 150mg	*Adult:* 50-200mg Q 12h.	C

Medication	Preparation	Dosing	Pregnancy Risk
Fluconazole (Diflucan)	Susp: 200mg/5ml Tab: 50, 100, 150, 200mg Inj: 2mg/ml	Child <13y.o.: **Oral/esophageal candidiasis:** 6mg/kg po/IV day 1, then 3mg/kg po/IV QD. **Systemic candidiasis:** 6-12mg/kg po/IV QD. **Cryptococcal meningitis:** 12mg/kg po/IV day 1, then 6mg/kg po/IV QD. Child >13y.o.-adult: **Oral/esophageal candidiasis:** start 200mg po/IV on day 1, then 100mg po/IV QD. Up to 400mg/d has been used. **Candida/yeast vaginitis:** 150mg po single dose. **Systemic candidiasis:** 400mg po/IV on day 1, then 200-800mg po/IV QD. **Cryptococcal meningitis:** 400mg po/IV on day 1, then 200-400mg po/IV QD.	C
Flucytosine (Ancobon)	Liquid: 10mg/ml (prepared by pharmacist) Cap: 250, 500mg	Child <1mo.: 50-100mg/kg QD or div BID. Child >1mo.-adult: 25-37.5mg/kg Q 6h.	C
Flumazenil (Romazicon)	Inj: 0.1mg/ml (5, 10ml)	**Reversal of benzodiazepines given for medical purposes:** Child: 0.01mg/kg (max 0.2mg); may repeat dose Q 1min as needed up to 5 doses. Adult: 0.2mg IV over 15sec. If no effect 45sec later, repeat same dose. May repeat at 1min intervals until total 1mg given.	C

	Suspected benzodiazepine OD: *Child:* same dosing as for child above. *Adult:* 0.2mg IV over 30sec. If no effect, try 0.3mg IV over 30sec. If still no effect, try 0.5mg IV over 30sec, then repeat Q 1min until total 3mg given.	C
Flunisolide (*AeroBid, Nasarel*)	*Inhaler:* 250μg/puff *Nasal spray:* 25μg/spray	**Inhaler:** *Child 6-15y.o.:* 2 puffs BID. *Child >15y.o.-adult:* 2-4 puffs BID. **Nasal spray:** *Child 6-15y.o.:* 2 sprays per nostril BID. *Child >15y.o.-adult:* 2 sprays per nostril BID-QID.	C
Fluorometholone ophthalmic (*FML, Fluor-Op*)	*Susp:* 0.1% in 5, 10ml *Forte:* Susp 0.25% *Ointment:* 0.1% in 3.5g	**Susp:** *Adult:* 1-2 drops BID-QID. Shake well before use. **Ointment:** apply 1/2 inch QD-TID.	C
Fluoxetine (*Prozac*)	*Liquid:* 20mg/5ml *Cap:* 10, 20, 40mg *Delayed-release cap:* 90mg	*Adult:* 20-80mg/d. Start at 20mg Qam. For larger doses, give two times/d with second dose at noon. Delayed-release cap: 90mg po Q wk.	C
Fluphenazine (*Prolixin*)	*Liquid:* 2.5mg/5ml; 5mg/5ml *Tab:* 1, 2.5, 5, 10mg *Inj:* 2.5mg/ml *Long acting inj:* 25mg/ml	**PO:** *Adult:* 2.5-10mg/d divided TID-QID, max 40mg/d. **IM:** *Adult:* 2.5-10mg/d divided Q 6-8h. **LA Inj:** *Adult:* 12.5-25mg IM Q 1-3wk.	C

Medication	Preparation	Dosing	Pregnancy Risk
Flurazepam *(Dalmane)*	*Cap:* 15, 30mg	*Adult:* 15-30mg hs prn.	X
Flurbiprofen *(Ansaid)*	*Tab:* 50, 100mg	*Adult:* 200-300mg/d, divided BID, TID, or QID; max 100mg/dose.	B,D3
Fluticasone *(Flovent, Flonase)*	*Inhaler:* 44, 110, 220μg/puff *Nasal spray:* 50μg/spray *Rotadisk:* 50, 100, 250μg *Diskus:* 50, 100, 250μg	**Inhaler:** *Child >12y.o.-adult:* 88-440μg BID. **Nasal spray:** *Child >4y.o.-adult:* 1 spray each nostril BID or 2 sprays each nostril QD. **Rotadisk/Diskus:** *Child 4-11y.o.:* start 50μg BID, titrate to max 100μg BID. *Child >11y.o.-adult:* start 100μg BID, max 500μg BID.	C
Fluvastatin *(Lescol)*	*Cap:* 20, 40mg *Cap XL:* 80mg	*Adult:* 20-80mg/d. Divide doses ≥40mg/d BID. Cap XL: 80mg po hs may be used in place of 40mg po BID dosing.	X
Fluvoxamine *(Luvox)*	*Tab:* 25, 50, 100mg	*Adult:* Start 50mg hs, increase as needed by 50mg every 4-7d. When dose >100mg/d divide BID, max 300mg/d.	C
Folic acid	*Tab:* 0.4, 0.8, 1.0mg *Inj:* 5mg/ml	*Folic acid deficiency: Child:* 1mg QD. *Adult:* 1mg QD. *Maintenance: Child <4y.o.:* 0.4mg QD. *Child >4y.o.- adult:* 0.5mg QD.	A,C§

Fondaparinux *(Arixtra)*	*Inj:* 2.5mg/0.5ml	*Adult:* DVT prophylaxis (hip/knee replacement) 2.5mg SC QD.	B
Formoterol *(Foradil)*	*Inh:* 12μg capsule for aerolizer	*>5y.o.-adult:* 1 cap aerolizer Q 12h; max 24μg/d.	C
Foscarnet *(Foscavir)*	*Inj:* 24mg/ml	***CMV retinitis:*** *Adult:* 60mg/kg IV over 1h Q 8h for 14-21d. **Herpes simplex:** *Adult:* 40mg/kg IV over 1h Q 8-12h for 14-21d.	C
Fosfomycin *(Monurol)*	*Powder for oral stln:* 3g	*Women ≥18y.o.:* ***Uncomplicated UTI:*** 3g po dissolved in water, single dose. ***Complicated UTI:*** 3g po QD for 3d.	B
Fosinopril *(Monopril)*	*Tab:* 10, 20, 40mg	*Adult:* start 10mg po QD, adjust by response, usual dose 20-40mg, max 80mg/d in single or divided doses.	C,D2-3
Fosphenytoin *(Cerebyx)*	*Inj:* 50PE/ml (PE = phenytoin equivalent)	*Child/adult:* ***Loading dose:*** 10-20PE/kg IM/IV (max rate 100-150PE/min IV). ***Maintenance:*** 4-6PE/kg QD IM/IV. *Dose as for phenytoin (formulated as phenytoin equivalent-PE).*	D
Frovatriptan *(Frova)*	*Tab:* 2.5mg	*Adult:* 2.5mg × 1, may repeat in 2h; max 7.5 mg/d.	C
Furazolidone *(Furoxone)*	*Liquid:* 50mg/15ml *Tab:* 100mg	***Giardiasis:*** see p. 109.	C

Medication	Preparation	Dosing	Pregnancy Risk
Furosemide (Lasix)	*Liquid:* 10mg/ml, 40mg/5ml *Tab:* 20, 40, 80mg *Inj:* 10mg/ml	**PO:** *Child:* initial 2mg/kg Q 6-12h; max 6mg/kg/d. *Adult:* start 20-80mg Q 12-24h. **IV:** *Child:* 1mg/kg. *Adult:* 40-60mg as initial Rx of CHF; double dose if no diuresis in 30min. Adjust dose upward for renal insufficiency or failure.	C,D(Htn)
Gabapentin (Neurontin)	*Tab:* 100, 200, 400, 600, 800mg	***Epilepsy:*** *Child 3-12y.o.:* 3-12mg/kg TID. *Child >12y.o.-adult:* 300-600mg po TID. ***P/herpetic neuralgia:*** *Adult:* 300mg single dose day 1, 300mg BID on day 2, 300mg TID on day 3, then titrated as needed to max 600mg TID.	C
Ganciclovir (Cytovene)	*Cap:* 250, 500mg *Inj:* 500mg	*Child >12y.o-adult:* **PO:** 1000mg TID with food. **IV:** 5mg/kg Q 12h for 14-21d, then 5mg/kg QD.	C
Gatifloxacin (Tequin)	*Inj:* 10mg/ml (20, 40ml) *Tab:* 200, 400mg	**PO/IV:** *Adult:* 400mg QD. *UTI:* 3d. ***Sinusitis:*** 10d. ***Bronchitis/complicated UTI/pyelonephritis:*** 7-10d. ***Community-acquired pneumonia:*** 7-14d. ***GC:*** 400mg single dose.	C

Gemfibrozil *(Lopid)*	*Tab:* 600mg *Cap:* 300mg	*Adult:* 600mg 30min before morning and evening meals.	C
Gemifloxacin *(Factive)*	*Tab:* 320mg	*Adult:* **Chronic bronchitis:** 320mg QD × 5d. **Community-acquired pneumonia:** 320mg × 7d. CrCl <40 mL/min and HD: 160mg QD.	C
Gentamicin *(Garamycin)*	*Inj:* 40mg/ml (adult); 10mg/ml (pediatric); 2mg/ml (intrathecal)	*Child <7d:* 2.5mg/kg IM/IV Q 12h. *Child >7d:* 2.5mg/kg (max 100mg) IM/IV Q 8h. *Adult:* load 2mg/kg IM/IV, then 1.7mg/kg Q 8h IM/IV. *Alternate QD dosing (only if adult <75y.o. with creat <1.5):* 4-7mg/kg QD IM/IV.	C
Gentamicin ophthalmic *(Garamycin)*	*Sltn:* 3mg/ml *Ointment:* 3mg/g	**Sltn:** *Adult:* 1-2 drops in affected eye Q 4h. In severe infections, the dosage may be increased to 2 drops Q 1h. **Ointment:** apply 1/2 inch to affected eye BID-TID.	C
Glimepiride *(Amaryl)*	*Tab:* 1, 2, 4mg	*Adult:* Start 1-2mg QD with breakfast, max 8mg QD.	C
Glipizide *(Glucotrol)*	*Tab regular:* 5, 10mg *Tab XL:* 2.5, 5, 10mg	*Adult:* <u>Tab regular:</u> start 2.5-5mg, adjust as needed up to 40 mg/d. When giving >15mg/d, divide BID. <u>Tab XL:</u> 5-20mg QD.	C

Medication	Preparation	Dosing	Pregnancy Risk
Glucagon	*Inj:* 1mg/ml	***Calcium channel blocker or beta-blocker*** *OD: Child:* 50μg/kg IV over 5min. *Adult:* 5-10mg IV over 1min. *See also pp. 57-58.*	B
Glyburide *(Micronase, DiaBeta, Glynase)*	*Tab:* 1.25, 2.5, 5mg *Glynase PresTab:* 1.5, 3, 4.5, 6mg	*Adult (tab):* 1.25-20mg QD. *Adult* (Glynase PresTab): 0.75-12mg QD. *Regular tab 5mg equivalent in potency to* Pres Tab 3mg.	C
Glyburide/ metformin *(Glucovance)*	*Tab:* G 1.25mg/M 250mg; G 2.5 mg/M 500mg; G 5mg/M 500mg	*Adult:* start G 1.25mg/M 250mg QD or BID with meals, adjust Q 2wk as needed to max G 20mg/M 2000mg/d.	C
Glycerin *(Osmoglyn)*	*Oral sltn:* 0.628g/ml (50%)	*Adult:* 2-3ml/kg. Give in chilled solution mixed with lemon juice.	C
Glycopyrrolate *(Robinul)*	*Tab:* 1, 2mg *Inj:* 0.2mg/ml	**PO:** *Child >12y.o.-adult:* 1-2mg BID-TID. **IV:** *Reversal of NM blockade: Child/adult:* 0.2mg per mg of neostigmine (or per 5mg of pyridostigmine) being administered simultaneously.	B
Granisetron *(Kytril)*	*Liquid:* 1mg *Tab:* 1mg *Inj:* 1mg	**PO:** *Adult:* 1mg po BID. **Inj:** *Adult:* 10μg/kg over 5min.	B

See index for proprietary names of generic meds

Griseofulvin *(Fulvicin, Griseactin, Grifulvin V)*	**Microsize:** *Tab:* 250, 500mg *Liquid:* 125mg/5ml **Ultramicrosize:** *Tab:* 125, 165, 250, 330mg	**Microsize:** *Child >2y.o.:* 5-10mg/kg QD or divided BID. *Adult:* 500-1000mg/d QD or divided BID. **Ultramicrosize:** *Child >2y.o.:* 7mg/kg QD. *Adult:* 330-750mg/d QD or divided BID. *Give all forms with fatty foods to avoid GI distress.*	C
Guanabenz *(Wytensin)*	*Tab:* 4, 8mg	*Adult:* 4-32mg Q 12h.	C
Guanfacine *(Tenex)*	*Tab:* 1, 2mg	*Adult:* 1-2mg hs.	B
Haloperidol *(Haldol)*	*Liquid:* 2mg/ml *Tab:* 0.5, 1, 2, 5, 10, 20mg *Inj:* 5, 50, 100mg/ml	**PO:** *Child 3-12y.o.:* 0.025-0.15mg/kg/d divided BID-TID. *Child >12y.o.-adult:* 2-5mg BID-TID. **IM:** *Child 6-12y.o.:* 1-3mg Q 4-8h, max 0.15mg/kg/d. *Child >12y.o.-adult:* 2-5mg Q 1h as needed.	C
Heparin	*Inj:* 10, 100, 1000, 2500, 5000, 7500, 10,000, 20,000, 40,000U/ml	**MI/unstable angina:** 60U/kg, then infusion at 12U/kg/h. **PE/DVT:** 80U/kg bolus, then infusion at 18U/kg/h. **See also: MI,** pp. 101-102; **PE,** pp. 132-133; **USA,** pp. 101-102; **DVT,** p. 143.	C

Medication	Preparation	Dosing						Pregnancy Risk
Hepatitis A vaccine	*Havrix:* 360ELU/0.5ml, 720ELU/0.5ml, 1440 ELU/ml *Vaqta:* 25U/0.5ml; 50U/ml	*Type of vaccine* Havrix Vaqta	*Age in y* 2-18 >18 2-17 ≥18	*Dose* 720ELU 1440ELU 25U 50U	*Schedule* 0, 6-12mo 0, 6-12mo 0, 6-18mo 0, 6mo			C
Hepatitis B immune globulin *(Hep-B-Gammagee, HyperHep, H-BIG)*	*Inj:* 0.5, 1, 5ml	*Neonates born to HBsAg-positive mothers:* 0.5ml IM at birth. *Child >1mo.-adult:* 0.06 ml/kg IM. Also give hepatitis B vaccine - see pp. 112-113.						C
Hepatitis B vaccine *(Recombivax HB, Engeri B)*	*Recombivax HB:* 5, 10, 30, 40μg/vial *Engerix-B:* 10, 20μg/vial	Post-exposure give hep B imm. globulin; also see pp. 112-113. Give IM in indicated doses at 0, 1, and 6mo. *Infants of HBsAg-pos mothers* *Other child <20y.o.* *Adults >20y.o.* *Dialysis/immuno-compromised adults** **Revaccinate if anti-HBS <10mlU >1-2mo. after 3rd dose.* *†Give this Engerix-B dose as two 20μg doses at different sites.*		*Recombivax HB* 5μg 2.5μg 10μg 40μg	*Engerix-B* 10μg 10μg 20μg 40μg†			B

204   *See index for proprietary names of generic meds*

Drug	Preparations	Dosage	Class
Homatropine ophthalmic *(Isopto Homatropine)*	*Sltn:* 2% and 5% in 5 and 15ml	***Uveitis:*** *Child:* use only 2%, 1-2 drops BID-TID and compress lacrimal sac by digital pressure for several min after instillation. *Adult:* 1-2 drops Q 3-4h.	C
Hydralazine *(Apresoline)*	*Tab:* 10, 25, 50, 100mg *Inj:* 20mg/ml	**PO:** *Child:* 0.2-1.8mg/kg Q 6h, max 25mg/dose. *Adult:* 10-50mg Q 6h. **IM/IV:** *Child:* 0.1-0.2mg/kg Q 4-6h, max 20mg/dose. *Adult:* 5-20mg IV Q 20min prn; 10-50mg IM Q 3-6h prn.	C
Hydrochlorothiazide *(Esidrix, HydroDIURIL)*	*Liquid:* 50mg/5ml *Tab:* 12.5, 25, 50, 100mg	*Child:* 1-2mg/kg/d QD or divided BID. *Adult:* 12.5-50mg/dose QD or BID.	B,D(Htn)
Hydrochlorothiazide/spironolactone *(Aldactazide)*	*Tab:* Hydro 25mg/Spiro 25mg; Hydro 50mg/Spiro 50mg	*Child:* as spironolactone, 1.65-3.3mg/kg/d QD or div BID. *Adult:* as spironolactone, 25-100mg/dose QD-BID.	C,D(Htn)
Hydrochlorothiazide/triamterene *(Dyazide, Maxzide)*	*Cap:* Hydro 25mg/Triam 37.5mg; Hydro 25mg/Triam 50mg; Hydro 50mg/Triam 75mg	*Adult:* 1-2 caps QD.	C, D (Htn)

Medication	Preparation	Dosing	Pregnancy Risk
Hydrocodone/ acetaminophen *(Vicodin, Vicodin ES)*	*Liquid:* Hy 2.5 mg/Acet 167mg per 5ml *Tab:* Hy 5, 7.5mg/Acet 325mg; Hy 2.5, 5, 7.5, 10mg/Acet 500mg; Hy 7.5, 10mg/Acet 650mg; Hy 10mg/Acet 660mg; Hy 7.5, 10mg/Acet 750mg	*Child:* as hydrocodone, 0.125mg/kg QID prn for pain. *Adult:* as hydrocodone, 5-10mg Q 4-6h prn for pain.	C
Hydrocodone/ ibuprofen *(Vicoprofen)*	*Tab:* Hy 7.5mg/Ibu 200mg	*Adult:* 1 tab Q 4-6h prn for pain.	C
Hydrocortisone *(Solu-Cortef)*	*Liquid:* 10mg/5ml *Tab:* 5, 10, 20mg *Inj:* 100, 250, 500, 1000mg/vial	*Dosage dependent on disease process being treated.*	C,D1
Hydroflumethi- azide *(Diucardin, Saluron)*	*Tab:* 50mg	**Diuresis:** *Adult:* 50mg QD-BID. **Hypertension:** *Adult:* 50mg BID.	C,D(Htn)

See index for proprietary names of generic meds

Hydromorphone *(Dilaudid)*	*Liquid:* 1mg/ml *Tab:* 2, 4, 8mg *Supp:* 3mg *Inj:* 1, 2, 4mg/ml	**IV/IM/SC:** *Child:* 0.015mg/kg Q 4-6h. *Adult:* 1-2mg Q 4-6h prn. **PO:** *Child:* 0.03-0.08 mg/kg Q 4-6h. *Adult:* 2-4mg Q 4h prn. **PR:** 1 supp Q 6-8h.	C,D(Htn)
Hydroxychloroquine *(Plaquenil)*	*Tab:* 200mg	*Adult:* **Lupus:** 200-800mg/d QD or divided BID. **Rheumatoid arthritis:** 200-600mg QD.	D
Hydroxyzine *(Atarax)* <u>po</u> *(Vistaril)* <u>IM</u>	*Liquid:* 10, 25mg/5ml *Tab:* 10, 25, 50, 100mg *Inj:* 25, 50mg/ml	**PO:** *Child:* 0.5mg/kg/d Q 6h prn. *Adult:* 25-100mg Q 6h prn. **IM:** *Child:* 0.5-1.0mg/kg Q 4-6h prn. *Adult:* 25-100mg Q 6h prn.	C
Ibandronate *(Bonviva)*	*Tab:* 2.5mg	*Adult:* 2.5mg QD.	C
Ibuprofen *(Motrin, Advil, Nuprin)*	*Liquid:* 100mg/2.5ml; 100mg/5ml *Oral drops:* 40mg/ml *Tab:* 50, 100, 200, 300, 400, 600, 800mg	*Child >6mo.:* 5-10mg/kg Q 6-8h. *Adult:* 200-800mg Q 6-8h.	D
Ibutilide *(Corvert)*	*Inj:* 0.1mg/ml	**IV:** *Adult <60kg:* 0.01mg/kg. *Adult ≥60kg:* 1mg. Give over 10min. May repeat dose 10min after initial dose complete.	B,D3

Medication	Preparation	Dosing	Pregnancy Risk
Idoxuridine ophthalmic *(Herplex)*	*Sltn:* 0.1% in 15ml	***Herpes simplex keratitis:*** *Adult:* 1 drop to infected eye Q 1h during the day, Q 2h at night. After healing has occurred, reduce to Q 2h during the day, Q 4h at night for an additional 3-7d.	C
Imipenem/cilastatin *(Primaxin I.V., Primaxin I.M.)*	*IV inj:* 250, 500mg/vial *IM inj:* 500, 750mg/vial	*Child >3mo.-3y.o.:* 25mg/kg IV Q 6h. *Child >3y.o.:* 12.5mg/kg IV Q 6h, max 4g/d. *Adult:* 0.25-1.0g IV Q 6-8h or 500-750mg IM Q 12h.	C
Imipramine *(Tofranil)*	*Tab:* 10, 25, 50mg	***Enuresis:*** *Child >6y.o.:* 25-75mg 1h before bedtime; max if <12y.o. is 50mg/dose. ***Depression:*** *Adult:* 100-300mg divided BID-TID.	D
Indapamide *(Lozol)*	*Tab:* 1.25, 2.5mg	*Adult:* **HTN:** 1.25-2.5mg QD. **Edema:** 2.5-5mg QD.	B,D(Htn)
Indinavir *(Crixivan)*	*Cap:* 100, 200, 333, 400mg	**PO:** *Child:* 500mg/m² Q 8h. *Adult:* 800mg Q 8h. Give on an empty stomach.	C
Indomethacin *(Indocin)*	*Liquid:* 25mg/5ml *Cap:* 25, 50mg *Cap (SR):* 75mg *Supp:* 50mg	***Gout attack, acute:*** p. 110. ***Other:*** *Child >14y.o.:* 1-3mg/kg/d divided TID or QID. *Adult:* 75-150mg/d po or PR divided TID-QID or SR 75mg po QD-BID.	D

See index for proprietary names of generic meds

Influenza virus, live *(FluMist)*	*Spray:* 0.5ml	*Child ≥5y.o.-adult:* 0.25ml/nostril intranasally. If 5-8y.o. and not previously given Flumist, repeat dose 6wk later.	C
Iodine *(Pima, SSKI)*	*PIMA:* 325mg/5ml *SSKI:* 1g/ml *Tab:* 130mg	**Thyrotoxicosis:** *Child <1y.o.:* 150-250mg (3-5 drops of SSKI) TID. *Child >1y.o.-adult:* 300-500mg (6-10 drops SSKI) TID.	D
Ipratropium bromide *(Atrovent)*	*Inhaler:* 18µg/puff *Inhltn sltn:* 0.5mg/vial *Nasal spray:* 21, 42µg/spray	**Inhaler:** *Adult:* 2 puffs QID. May be taken more frequently as needed, not to exceed 12 puffs/24h. **Nebulized:** *Adult:* 0.5mg in 2.5ml NS Q 6-8h. **Nasal spray:** 21µg/spray twice BID-TID or 42µg/spray twice TID-QID.	B
Irbesartan *(Avapro)*	*Tab:* 75, 150, 300mg	**HTN:** *Adult:* 150-300mg QD.	C, D2-3
Isocarboxazid *(Marplan)*	*Tab:* 10mg	*Adult:* start 10mg BID, then titrate to lowest effective dose, usually 10-60mg/d.	C
Isoetharine *(Bronkosol)*	*Inhalation solution:* multiple concentrations	**Inhaler:** *Adult:* 1-2 puffs Q 3-4h. **Nebulized:** *Child:* 0.1-0.2mg/kg (max 5mg) with 2ml NS Q 2-6h. *Adult:* 5mg with 2ml NS nebulized Q 2-6h.	C

Medication	Preparation	Dosing	Pregnancy Risk
Isoniazid (INH)	*Liquid:* 50mg/5ml *Tab:* 50, 100, 300mg *Inj:* 100mg/ml	***Daily TB Rx/prophylaxis:*** *Child:* 10-15mg/kg (max 300mg) QD. *Adult:* 300mg QD. ***Twice weekly TB Rx:*** *Child:* 20-40mg/kg (max 900mg). *Adult:* 15mg/kg (max 900mg).	C
Isoproterenol *(Isuprel)*	*Inhaler:* 131µg/puff *Inhalation sltn:* 0.25%, 0.5%, 1% *Inj:* 0.2mg/ml	**Inhaler:** *Child/adult:* 1-2 puffs Q 4h prn. **Nebulized:** *Child:* 0.05mg/kg (min 0.5mg, max 1.25mg) diluted with 2ml NS Q 4h. *Adult:* 2.5-5.0mg dilute with 2ml NS Q 4h. **IV: Heart block:** *Child:* start 0.05µg/kg/min, titrate to max 2µg/kg/min infusion. *Adult:* start 2µg/min, titrate to max 20µg/min infusion.	C
Isosorbide dinitrate *(Isordil, Sorbitrate, Dilatrate-SR)*	*Sublingual tab:* 2.5, 5, 10mg *Tab (chew):* 5, 10mg (Sorbitrate) *Tab:* 5, 10, 20, 30, 40mg *Cap/Tab (LA):* 40mg (scored) (Isordil) (Dilatrate-SR)	*Adult:* Sublingual or chew tab: 2.5-10mg Q 5min prn for pain or before activity likely to cause angina. <u>Tab:</u> 5-40mg Q 6h. <u>LA tab:</u> 40-80mg Q 8-12h. *Use smallest effective dose.*	C
Isoxsuprine *(Vasodilan)*	*Tab:* 10, 20mg	*Adult:* 10-20mg TID-QID.	C

See index for proprietary names of generic meds

Isradipine *(DynaCirc)*	*Cap:* 2.5, 5mg *Tab SR:* 5, 10mg	*Adult:* 2.5-10mg BID. *Tab SR:* 5-20mg QD.	C
Itraconazole *(Sporanox)*	*Liquid:* 100mg/10ml *Cap:* 100mg *Inj:* 250mg	*Adult:* **PO:** 200mg QD with food. Increase in 100mg increments to max 400mg/d. If giving more than 200mg/d, divide BID. **IV:** 200mg Q 12h for 4 doses, then 200mg QD.	C
Kayexalate **(Sodium polystyrene sulfonate)**	*Liquid:* 15g/60ml *Powder:* 3.5g/5ml	*Child:* 1g/kg po or as retention enema Q 2-6h. *Adult:* 15-60g po or 30-50g as retention enema Q 2-6h.	C
Ketamine *(Ketalar)*	*Inj:* 10, 50, 100mg/ml	***Sedation for rapid-sequence intubation:*** *Child/adult:* 1-4.5mg/kg over 60sec IV. See pp. 15-16 for RSI protocol.	B
Ketoconazole *(Nizoral)*	*Tab:* 200mg *Cream:* 2% *Shampoo:* 1%, 2%	**Tab:** *Child* >2y.o.: 3.3-6.6mg/kg QD. *Adult:* 200-400mg QD. **Cream:** Apply QD-BID for 2wk. **Shampoo:** Apply twice/wk for 4wk. *Applications should be ≥3d apart.*	C
Ketoprofen *(Orudis, Oruvail SR)*	*Tab:* 12.5 (OTC), 25, 50, 75mg *Tab SR:* 100, 150, 200mg	**Analgesia:** *Adult:* 25-75mg TID-QID. **Rheumatoid/osteoarthritis:** *Adult:* start 75mg po TID or 50mg QID, max 300mg/d. Tab SR: 200mg QD.	B,D3

Medication	Preparation	Dosing	Pregnancy Risk
Ketorolac (*Toradol*)	*Tab:* 10mg *Inj:* 15, 30, 60mg/ml	*Adult:* **PO:** 10mg Q 4-6h prn (max 40mg/d for max 5d). **IM:** initial 30-60mg; then 15-30mg Q 6h prn (max 120mg/d for max 5d). *Elderly (>65y), renal insuff, or wt <50kg:* 30mg, then 15mg Q 6h (max 60mg/d for max 5d). **IV:** initial 30mg; then 15-30mg Q 6h prn (max 120mg/d for max 5d). *Elderly (>65y), renal insuff, or wt <50kg:* 15mg Q 6h (max 60 mg/d for max 5d).	C,D3
Ketorolac ophthalmic (*Acular*)	*Sltn:* 0.5% in 3, 5, 10ml	*Adult:* 1 drop QID.	C,D3
Ketotifen opthalmic (*Zaditor*)	*Sltn:* 0.025%	*Adult:* 1 drop in affected eye Q 8-12h.	C
Labetalol (*Trandate, Normodyne*)	*Tab:* 100, 200, 300mg *Inj:* 5mg/ml (20, 40ml)	**PO:** *Child:* start at 4mg/kg/d, titrate to max 40mg/kg/d divided BID. *Adult:* usual 100-400mg BID. Max 2.4g/d divided TID. **IV intermittent dosing:** *Child:* 0.3-1.0mg/kg (max 20mg) Q 10min prn. *Adult:* 20mg over 2min, then 40-80mg Q 10min, max total 300mg. **IV infusion for hypertensive emergency:** *Child:* Start 0.4-1.0mg/kg/h, titrate to max 3mg/kg/h. Loading dose of 0.2-1.0mg/kg (max 20mg) may be given before infusion. *Adult:* start 2mg/min, titrate. Max total 300mg.	C,D2-3

Lactulose *(Cephulac, Duphalac)*	*Liquid:* 10g/15ml	**Constipation:** *Child:* 7.5ml po after break-fast. *Adult:* start 15-30ml po QD, may titrate to 60ml po QD as needed. **Hepatic encephalopathy: PO:** 30-45ml TID-QID. Adjust dose to obtain 2-3 loose stools/d. **PR:** retention enema with 300ml diluted with 700ml of NS. Retain for 30-60min Q 4-6h.	B
Lamivudine *(Epivir, 3TC)*	*Liquid:* 5, 10mg/ml *Tab:* 100, 150mg	**HIV:** *Child 3mo.-16y.o.:* 4mg/kg (max 150mg) BID. *Child 16y.o.-adult <50kg:* 2mg/kg (max 150mg) BID. *Child 16y.o.-adult >50kg:* 150mg BID. **Chronic hepatitis B:** *Child 2-17y.o.:* 3mg/kg, max 100mg QD. *Adult:* 100mg QD.	C
Lamivudine/ zidovudine *(Combivir)*	*Tab:* Lamivudine 150mg/Zidovudine 300mg	*Child >12y.o.-adult:* 1 tab BID.	C
Lamotrigine *(Lamictal)*	*Tab:* 25, 50, 100, 150, 200mg *Chew tab:* 5, 25mg	**Usual maintenance on other anticonvul-sants but not valproate:** *Child 2-12y.o.:* 2.5-7.5mg/kg BID. *Child >12y.o.-adult:* 150-250mg po BID. **Usual maintenance on other anticonvul-sants, including valproate:** *Child 2-12y.o.:* 1-5mg/kg QD or divided BID. *Child >12y.o.-adult:* 100-400mg po QD or divided BID.	C

Medication	Preparation	Dosing	Pregnancy Risk
Lansoprazole *(Prevacid)*	*Cap:* 15, 30mg	***Duodenal ulcer:*** 15mg QD for 4wk. ***Gastric ulcer:*** 30mg QD for 8wk. ***Erosive esophagitis:*** 30mg QD for up to 8wk. ***Hypersecretory conditions:*** Up to 180mg QD-BID, titrated to reduce acid secretion to <10mEq/h.	B
Latanoprost ophthalmic *(Xalatan)*	*Sltn:* 0.005% in 2.5ml	***IOP:*** *Adult:* 1 drop in affected eye QD hs.	C
Lepirudin *(Refludan)*	*Inj:* 50mg/vial	*Adult:* 0.4mg/kg slowly IV, max 44mg; then 0.15mg/kg/h, max 16.5mg/h.	B
Letrozole *(Femara)*	*Tab:* 2.5mg	*Adult female:* ***Breast CA:*** 2.5mg QD.	D
Levalbuterol *(Xopenex)*	*Inhalation sltn:* 0.31, 0.63, 1.25mg	*Child 12y.o.-adult:* 0.63-1.25mg nebulized Q 6-8h.	C B
Levobunolol ophthalmic *(Betagan, AKBeta)*	*Sltn:* 0.25% in 5 and 10ml; 0.5% in 5, 10, and 15ml	***Glaucoma:*** *Adult:* 1 drop in affected eye QD or BID.	C
Levocabastine ophthalmic *(Livostin)*	*Susp:* 0.05% in 5 and 10ml	***Allergic conjunctivitis:*** *Adult:* 1 drop QID.	C

See index for proprietary names of generic meds

Levodopa (*L-dopa, Larodopa, Dopar*)	*Tab:* 100, 250, 500mg *Cap:* 100, 250, 500mg	*Adult:* start 0.5-1.0g/d, divided BID, TID, or QID with food. May increase by up to 0.75g/d every 3-7d to max 8g/d. *Usually given in combination with carbidopa as Sinemet - see below.*	C
Levodopa/ carbidopa (*Sinemet*)	*Tab:* Lev 100mg/Carb 10mg (<u>Sinemet 10-100</u>); Lev 100mg/ Carb 25mg (<u>Sinemet 25-100</u>); Lev 250mg/ Carb 25mg (<u>Sinemet 25-250</u>) *Tab SR:* Lev 100mg/ Carb 25mg (<u>Sinemet CR 25-100</u>); Lev 200mg/Carb 50mg (<u>Sinemet CR 50-200</u>)	*Adult:* usual starting dose 1 tab <u>Sinemet 25-100</u> TID. Increase dose by 1 tab/d <u>Sinemet 25-100</u> every 1-2d to obtain desired effect (max 200/800 mg/d). Usual maintenance dose of carbidopa is 70-100 mg/d. *Tab SR:* usual starting dose 1 tab <u>Sinemet CR 50-200</u> BID, titrated to usual dose of levodopa 400-1600mg/d, rarely as high as 2400mg/d. *Special recommendations apply for titrating dosing and for transferring patients to SR tab from other levodopa regimens.*	C
Levofloxacin (*Levaquin*)	*Tab:* 250, 500, 750mg *Inj:* 25mg/ml *Inj:* 5mg/ml (in D5W)	*Adult:* **COPD:** 500mg QD × 7d. **Community-acquired pneumonia:** 500mg QD 7-14d. **Skin infection:** 500mg QD 10-14d. **UTI (including pyelo):** 250mg QD × 10d. *Dosing noted applies to po and IV routes.*	C
Levorphanol (*Levo-Dromoran*)	*Tab:* 2mg *Inj:* 2mg/ml	*Adult:* **PO/SC:** 2mg. May increase to 3mg if necessary.	D

Medication	Preparation	Dosing	Pregnancy Risk
Levothyroxine (**Synthroid**, **Levothroid**, **Levoxyl**)	*Tab:* 25, 50, 75, 88, 100, 112, 125, 137, 150, 175, 200, 300µg *Inj:* 200, 500µg	**IV doses are half of the following PO dosing:** *Maintenance: Child <6mo.:* 8-10µg/kg QD. *Child 6-12mo.:* 6-8µg/kg QD. *Child 1-5y.o.:* 5-6µg/kg QD. *Child 6-12y.o.:* 4-5µg/kg QD. *Child >12y.o.:* 2-3µg/kg QD. *Adult:* 100-200µg QD. *New dx hypothyroidism:* start 12.5-50µg/d, may increase by 25-50µg/d Q 2-4wk until desired effect obtained. *Hypothyroid coma:* see p. 117.	A
Lidocaine (**Xylocaine**)	*Inj:* 10, 20, 40, 100, 200mg/ml *Viscous oral sltn:* 2% (2g/100ml)	*VF/VT: Children:* 1mg/kg IV. May repeat in 5-10min, then start 10-50µg/kg/min infusion. *Adult:* 1-1.5mg/kg (1.5mg/kg if cardiac arrest) IV. If no effect, repeat 0.5-0.75mg/kg Q 5-10min, max 3mg/kg over 1h. If successful, infusion at 1-4mg/min. Repeat 0.5mg/kg bolus if recurrent VF/VT, then adjust infusion rate. *ET dose = 2-2.5 times IV dose. Reduce all doses by 50% for CHF, shock, or if age >70y.o.* *Oral topical anesthesia: Children/adult:* 15ml swish and spit/swallow Q 3-8h as needed.	B

See index for proprietary names of generic meds

Lindane (Gamma benzene hexachloride) (Kwell)	*Lotion, shampoo:* 1%	*Lice:* see p. 117. *Scabies:* see p. 133.	C
Linezolid (Zyvox)	*Powder for oral susp.:* 20mg/ml *Tab:* 400, 600mg *Inj:* 200, 400, 600mg	*Adult:* 600mg IV Q 12h or 400-600mg po Q 12h.	C
Liothyronine (Cytomel, Triostat)	*Tab:* 5, 25, 50µg *Inj:* 10µg/ml	*Adult:* usual maintenance 25-75µg QD. To initiate Rx, start 25µg QD. May increase by 12.5-25µg/dose Q 1-2wk.	A
Lisinopril (Prinivil, Zestril)	*Tab:* 2.5, 5, 10, 20, 40mg	*Adult <65y.o.:* start 10mg QD. Increase by 5-10mg/d Q 1-2wk. *Adult ≥65y.o.:* start 2.5-5 mg/d. Increase by 2.5-5mg/d Q 1-2wk. *Usual dose range 20-40mg/d.* **AMI (hemodynamically stable):** 5mg po stat, then 5mg po at 24h, 10mg at 48h, then 10mg po QD for 6wk. *For all indications adjust for renal insufficiency.*	C,D2-3
Lithium (Eskalith, Lithobid, Lithotabs, Lithonate)	*Liquid:* 300mg/5ml *Tab/Cap:* 150, 300, 600mg *Tab (SR):* 300mg (Lithobid), 450mg (Eskalith CR)	**Maintenance:** *Child:* 15-60mg/kg/d (max 2400mg/d). *Adult:* 900-2400mg/d. *Divide as follows: liquid, tab, cap: TID-QID; Eskalith CR: BID; Lithobid: BID-TID.*	D

Medication	Preparation	Dosing	Pregnancy Risk
Lomefloxacin (*Maxaquin*)	*Tab:* 400mg	*Adult:* **UTI, lower resp infection:** 400mg QD for 3-14d (UTI) or 10d (lower resp infection).	C
Loperamide (*Imodium*)	*Liquid:* 1mg/5ml *Cap:* 2mg *Tab:* 2mg	*Child 2-6y.o. (13-20kg):* 1mg TID on day 1. *Child 6-8y.o. (20-30kg):* 2mg BID on day 1. *Child 9-12y.o. (>30kg):* 2mg TID on day 1. *Children 2-12y.o.: After day 1, give 0.1mg/kg (but not more than the initial dose) after each unformed stool.* *Child >12y.o.-adult:* start 4mg, then give 2mg after each unformed stool (max 16mg/d).	B
Loracarbef (2nd-gen) (*Lorabid*)	*Liquid:* 100mg/5ml, 200mg/5ml *Cap:* 200, 400mg	*Child:* **Acute OM:** 15mg/kg (max 400mg) Q 12h for 10d. **Pharyngitis:** 15mg/kg (max 400mg) Q 12h for 10d. *Adult:* **Resp infection:** 200-400mg Q 12h for 10d (lower) or 10-14d (upper). **Skin/soft tissue:** 200mg Q 12h for 7d. **Lower UTI:** 200mg po QD for 7d. **Pyelonephritis, uncompromised pt:** 400mg Q 12h for 14d.	B
Loratadine (*Claritin*)	*Liquid:* 1mg/ml *Tab:* 10mg	*Child 2-5y.o.:* 5mg QOD. *Child >6y.o.-adult:* 10mg QD on an empty stomach.	B

See index for proprietary names of generic meds

Lorazepam (*Ativan*)	*Liquid:* 2, 4mg/ml *Tab:* 0.5, 1, 2mg *Inj:* 2, 4mg/ml	**PO:** *Child:* 0.05mg/kg Q 8h. *Adult:* 1-10mg/d div BID-TID. **IV:** **Sedation:** *Child:* 0.05mg/kg (max 4mg). *Adult:* 2-4mg/dose. **Alcohol withdrawal:** see p. 93. **Status epilepticus:** see pp. 136-137.	D
Losartan (*Cozaar*)	*Tab:* 25, 50, 100mg	**HTN:** start 25-100mg QD-BID, then adjust Q wk.	C,D2-3
Loteprednol ophthalmic (*Alrex, Lotemax*)	*Sltn:* 0.2%, 0.5%	*Adult:* 1-2 drops QID.	C
Lovastatin (*Mevacor, Altocor*)	*Tab:* 10, 20, 40mg *Tab ER:* 10, 20, 40, 60mg	*Adult:* start 20mg (or 40mg for extremely high cholesterol) with dinner. Increase dose Q 4wk until desired effect. Max 80mg/d in single or divided doses. Tab ER (*Altocor*): 10-60mg QD.	X
Loxapine (*Loxitane*)	*Liquid:* 25mg/ml *Cap:* 5, 10, 25, 50mg *Inj:* 50mg/ml	**PO:** *Adult:* 10-50mg BID. **IM:** *Adult:* 12.5-50mg Q 4-6h prn.	C
Magnesium citrate	*Liquid:* 300ml/bottle	*Child <6y.o.:* 0.5ml/kg, max 200ml QD. *Child 6-12y.o.:* 100-150ml QD. *Child >12y.o.-adult:* 100-300ml QD, usual dose 240ml.	A

Medication	Preparation	Dosing	Pregnancy Risk
Magnesium sulfate	*Inj:* 100, 125, 250, 500mg/ml (0.8, 1, 2, 4mEq/ml)	***Cardiac arrest/torsades:*** 2g IVP. ***Torsades/no cardiac arrest:*** 2g IV over 5-60min, infusion 0.5-1g/h. ***Hypomagnesemia:*** *Child/adult:* 25-50mg/kg IM/IV Q 4-6h. *Larger doses for severe cases.* ***Eclampsia:*** see p. 105.	B
Mannitol *(Osmitrol, Resectisol)*	*Inj:* 5%, 10%, 15%, 20%, 25%	***Intracranial pressure:*** *Child/adult:* initial dose 0.5-1g/kg IV, then 0.25-0.5g/kg IV as needed.	C
Maprotiline *(Ludiomil)*	*Tab:* 25, 50, 75mg	*Adult:* 25-150mg QD or in divided doses. In some severely depressed patients, up to 225mg/d may be given.	B
Mebendazole *(Vermox)*	*Tab (chew):* 100mg	***Worms:*** see pp. 143-144.	C
Meclizine *(Antivert)*	*Tab:* 12.5, 25, 50mg *Cap:* 25mg *Tab (chew):* 25mg	*Child >12y.o.-adult:* ***Vertigo:*** 25-100mg/d divided Q 6-12h. ***Motion sickness:*** 25-50mg 1h before departure, may repeat QD.	B
Meclofenamate *(Meclomen)*	*Cap:* 50, 100mg	*Child >14y.o.-adult:* 50-100mg Q 4-6h.	B,D3
Mefenamic acid *(Ponstel)*	*Cap:* 250mg	*Child >14y.o.-adult:* 500mg, then 250mg Q 6h for up to 1wk.	C
Mefloquine *(Lariam)*	*Tab:* 250mg	See pp. 119-120.	C,D3

See index for proprietary names of generic meds

Megestrol acetate (Megace)	Liquid: 40mg/ml Tab: 20, 40mg	HIV with cachexia: as liquid, 800mg QD. Breast CA: 40mg QID. Endometrial CA: 40-320mg/d in divided doses.	D
Memantine (Namenda)	Tab: 5, 10mg	Alzheimer's: Adult: start 5mg QD for 1wk, then 5mg BID for 1wk, then 10mg AM and 5mg PM for 1wk, then 10mg BID.	B
Meperidine (Demerol)	Liquid: 50mg/5ml Tab: 50, 100mg Inj: 25, 50, 75, 100mg/ml	PO/SC/IM/IV: Child: 1.0-1.5mg/kg Q 3-4h, max 100mg/dose. Adult: 50-150mg Q 3-4h prn.	D
Meropenem (Merrem)	Inj: 0.5, 1.0g	Intraabdominal infections: Child <50kg: 20mg/kg IV Q 8h. Child >50kg: 1g IV Q 8h. Adult: 1g IV Q 8h. Meningitis: Child <50kg: 40mg/kg IV Q 8h. Child >50kg-adult: 2g IV Q 8h.	B
Mesalamine (Asacol, Pentasa, Rowasa)	Cap (Pentasa): 250mg Supp (Rowasa): 500mg Tab (Asacol): 400mg Susp for enema (Rowasa): 4g/60ml	Ulcerative colitis: PO: Cap: 1g QID. Tab: 800mg TID. PR: Supp: 500mg Q 12h. Retention enema: 60ml (4g) hs, retain overnight (approx 8h). Usual course of therapy is 3-6wk.	B
Mesoridazine (Serentil)	Liquid: 25mg/ml Tab: 10, 25, 50, 100mg Inj: 25mg/ml	PO: Adult: Dose range is 30mg-400mg/d, divided BID-TID, depending on entity under treatment. IM: Adult: 25mg, may repeat in 30-60min.	C

Medication	Preparation	Dosing	Pregnancy Risk
Metaproterenol *(Alupent)*	*Liquid:* 10mg/5ml *Tab:* 10, 20mg *Inhaler:* 650µg/puff *Inhalation sltn:* 0.4%, 0.65%	**PO:** *Child <2y.o.:* 0.4mg/kg Q 8-12h. *Child 2-6y.o.:* 1.3-2.6mg/kg/d divided Q 6-8h. *Child 6-9y.o.:* 10mg Q 6-8h. *Child >9y.o.-adult:* 20mg Q 6-8h. **Inhaler:** *Child/adult:* 2-3 puffs Q 3-4h; max 12 puffs/d. **Nebulized:** *Child:* 0.01-0.02ml/kg of 5% sltn Q 4-6h. *Adult:* 0.3ml of 5% sltn Q 4-6h.	C
Metformin *(Glucophage)*	*Liquid:* 100mg/ml *Tab:* 500, 850, 1000mg *Tab ER:* 500, 750mg	*Child 10-16y.o.:* start 500mg BID with meals. Increase Q wk by 500 mg/d, max 2000mg/d. *Child 17y.o.-adult:* start 500mg BID or 850mg QD. Increase (1) if 500mg, by 500mg Q week, (2) if 850mg tabs, by 850mg every other week, (3) if liquid, by 500mg each BID dose every other week. For doses >2000mg/d, divide TID. Max dose = 2550mg. Tab ER: start 500mg with dinner, increase Q wk by 500mg max.	B
Methadone *(Dolophine)*	*Liquid:* 5, 10mg/5ml, 10mg/ml *Tab:* 5, 10, 40mg *Inj:* 10mg/ml	***Analgesia:*** 2.5-10mg po/SC/IM Q 3-4h prn. ***Detox:*** start 40-180mg/d, taper over not more than 21d. ***Maintenance of drug-free state:*** 15-120mg/d.	D

See index for proprietary names of generic meds

Drug	Form	Dosage	
Methazolamide *(Neptazane)*	*Tab:* 25, 50mg	***Glaucoma:*** *Adult:* 50-100mg BID-TID. ***Mountain sickness:*** 150-200mg QD. ***Essential tremor:*** 50-75mg QD.	C
Methenamine hippurate *(Hiprex, Urex)*	*Tab:* 1g (scored)	*Child 6-12y.o.:* 12.5-25mg/kg (max 1g) Q 12h. *Child >12y.o.-adult:* 1g Q 12h.	C
Methenamine mandelate *(Mandelamine)*	*Liquid:* 200 or 500mg/5ml *Tab:* 500, 1000mg	*Child 6-12y.o.:* 12-18mg/kg (max 1g) Q 6h. *Child 12y.o.-adult:* 1g po QID after meals and hs.	C
Methenamine/ phenyl salicylate/ atropine/ hyoscyamine/ benzoic acid/ methylene blue *(Urised)*	*Tab:* Meth 40.8mg/ Phen 18.1mg/Atro 0.03mg/Hyos 0.03mg	*Adult:* 2 tabs Q 6h.	C
Methimazole *(Tapazole)*	*Tab:* 5, 10mg	*Child:* start 0.4-0.7mg/kg/d div TID to control hyperthyroidism. *Max dose 30mg/d, maintenance ¹/₂ of initial dose.* *Adult:* start 5-20mg Q 8h, dose depending on severity of hyperthyroidism. *Maintenance ¹/₂ of initial dose.*	D

Medication	Preparation	Dosing	Pregnancy Risk
Methocarbamol (*Robaxin*)	*Tab:* 500, 750mg *Inj:* 100mg/ml	*Child >16y.o.-adult:* **PO:** 1500mg QID for 2-3d, then 4-4.5g/d div. 3-6 times/d. **IM/IV:** 1000mg Q 8h. Do not use >3 consecutive d. *Max IM:* 500mg/site.	C
Methsuximide (*Celontin*)	*Cap:* 150, 300mg	*Child:* 3.75-10mg/kg Q 6-8h. *Adult:* 300mg Q 6-12h.	C
Methyclothiazide (*Enduron*)	*Tab:* 2.5, 5mg	*Child:* 0.05-0.2mg/kg, max 10mg QD. *Adult:* 2.5-10mg QD.	B
Methyldopa (*Aldomet*)	*Liquid:* 250mg/5ml *Tab:* 125, 250, 500mg *Inj:* 50mg/ml	**PO:** *Child:* 10-65mg/kg/d divided Q 6-12h, max 3g/d. *Adult:* 500mg-3.0g/d divided BID-QID. **IV:** *Child:* 2-10mg/kg Q 6-8h (max 65mg/kg/d or 3g/d, whichever is less). *Adult:* 250-1000mg Q 6h.	B
Methylene blue	*Inj:* 10mg/ml	*Child/adult:* 1-2mg/kg IV over 5min, repeat in 1h prn.	C
Methylprednisolone (*Medrol, Solu-Medrol*)	*Tab:* 2, 4, 8, 16, 24, 32mg *Inj:* 40-2000mg/vial	*Dosage dependent on disease process being treated.*	NR
Methysergide (*Sansert*)	*Tab:* 2mg	*Migraine or vascular headache: Adult:* 4-8mg/d divided TID with meals. *Max duration of use is for 6mo.*	X
Metipranolol ophthalmic (*OptiPranolol*)	*Sltn:* 0.3% in 5 or 10ml	*Glaucoma: Adult:* 1 drop in affected eye BID.	C

See index for proprietary names of generic meds

Drug	Forms	Dosage	Category
Metoclopramide (*Reglan*)	*Liquid:* 5, 10mg/5ml *Tab:* 5, 10mg *Inj:* 5mg/ml	**GERD:** *Child:* 0.1-0.2mg/kg po Q 6-8h. *Adult:* 10-15mg po QID 30min before meals and hs. **Diabetic gastroparesis:** *Child:* 0.1-0.2mg/kg po/IM/IV Q 6-8h. *Adult:* 10mg po QID 30min before meals and hs or 10mg IM/IV Q 4-6h prn.	B
Metocurine iodide (*Metubine Iodide*)	*Inj:* 2mg/ml	*Adult:* 0.2-0.4mg/kg IV over 30-60sec.	C
Metolazone (*Zaroxolyn, Diulo Mykrox*)	*Tab:* 2.5, 5, 10mg *Tab (prompt release):* 0.5mg	*Child:* 0.2-0.4mg/kg QD. *Adult:* 2.5-20mg QD. *Prompt-release tab:* 0.5-1mg QD.	B,D(Htn)
Metoprolol (*Lopressor, Toprol XL*)	*Tab:* 50, 100mg *Tab (XL):* 25, 50, 100, 200mg *Inj:* 1mg/ml	**HTN:** *Adult:* 100-450mg/d po QD or divided BID. <u>Tab XL</u>: 50-400mg po QD. **Angina:** *Adult:* 50-200mg po BID. <u>Tab XL</u>: 100-400mg po QD. **MI:** see pp. 101-102.	C,D2-3
Metronidazole (*Flagyl, Protostat*)	*Cap:* 375mg *Tab:* 250, 500mg *Tab ER:* 750mg *Gel:* 0.75% in vag applicator (total 5g/dose) *Inj:* 500mg	**PO: Giardia:** p. 109. **Trichomonas:** p. 142. **Bact. vaginosis:** p. 141. **IV:** *Child >1mo.-adult:* initial dose 15mg/kg, then 7.5mg/kg (max 1g) Q 6h.	B
Mexiletine (*Mexitil*)	*Cap:* 150, 200, 250mg	*Adult:* 200-400mg Q 8h.	C

Medication	Preparation	Dosing	Pregnancy Risk
Mezlocillin (*Mezlin*)	*Inj:* 1, 2, 3, 4g	*Child <7d:* 75mg/kg IM/IV Q 12h. *Child >7d:* 75mg/kg IM/IV. *If ≤2kg, give Q 8h; if >2kg, give Q 6h.* *Adult:* 1.5-4g IM/IV Q 4-6h, max 24g/d.	B
Miconazole (*Monistat 3, Monistat 7*)	*Vag supp:* 100, 200mg *Cream/lotion:* 2%, 4%	**Vaginal candidiasis:** vag supp in vagina hs for 3d (*Monistat 3* 200mg) or 7d (*Monistat 7* 100mg). **Tinea corporis, tinea cruris, or tinea pedis and cutaneous candidiasis:** apply cream or lotion BID for 2-4wk.	C
Midazolam (*Versed*)	*Liquid:* 2mg/ml *Inj:* 1 or 5mg/ml	**Procedure sedation: PO:** *Child >6mo:* 0.25-0.5mg/kg 30min prior, max 20mg. *Child <6mo. may require up to 1mg/kg.* **IV:** *Child 6mo.-5y.o.:* 0.05-0.1mg/kg over 2-3min. May repeat Q 2-3min to max total 0.6mg/kg or 6mg total. *Child 6-12y.o.:* 0.025-0.05mg/kg over 2-3min. May repeat Q 2-3min to max total 0.4mg/kg or 10mg total. *Child >12y.o.-adult:* 0.5-2mg over 2-3min. May repeat Q 2-3min to usual max total 5-10mg. *For elderly patients, start with 1mg.*	D

See index for proprietary names of generic meds

Milrinone *(Primacor)*	*Inj:* 1mg/ml	**CHF loading dose:** *Adult:* 50µg/kg IV over 10min. **CHF maintenance infusion:** *Adult:* 0.375-0.75µg/kg/min IV. Total dose/d = 0.59-1.13mg/kg.	C
Minocycline *(Minocin)*	*Liquid:* 50mg/5ml *Tab/cap:* 50, 100mg *Inj:* 100mg	**PO/IV:** *Child* >8y.o.: initial dose 4mg/kg (max 200mg), then 2mg/kg (max 100mg) Q 12h. *Adult:* first dose 200mg, then 100mg Q 12h.	D
Minoxidil *(Loniten)*	*Tab:* 2.5, 10mg	*Child* <12y.o.: start 0.2mg/kg (max 5mg) QD. Usual dose 0.25-1.0mg/kg/d divided QD-BID, max 50mg/d. *Child* >12y.o.adult: usual effective dose 5-40mg/d po divided QD-BID, max 100mg/d.	C
Mirtazapine *(Remeron)*	*Tab:* 15, 30, 45mg *Solutab:* 15, 30, 45mg	*Adult:* Initial dose 15mg nightly; titrate up to 15-45mg/d. Increase no more frequently than Q 1-2wk.	C
Misoprostol *(Cytotec)*	*Tab:* 100, 200µg	*Adult:* 100-200µg QID or 400µg BID with food.	X
Mivacurium *(Mivacron)*	*Inj:* 0.5mg/ml; 2mg/ml	*Child* 2-12y.o.: 0.2mg/kg IV. **IV infusion:** 5-31µg/kg/min. *Adult:* 0.15-0.25mg/kg IV. **IV infusion:** 1-15µg/kg/min. *Dose should be based on lean body weight.*	C
Moexipril *(Univasc)*	*Tab:* 7.5, 15mg	*Adult:* start 7.5mg QD 1h before eating, titrate to up to 30mg/d in 1-2 doses 1h before meals.	C,D2-3

Medication	Preparation	Dosing	Pregnancy Risk
Mometasone *(Nasonex)*	*Spray:* 50µg/spray	**Allergic rhinitis:** *Child 3-11y.o.:* 1 spray/nostril QD. *Child 11y.o.-adult:* 2 sprays each nostril QD.	C
Montelukast *(Singulair)*	*Tab chew:* 4, 5mg *Tab:* 10mg	*Child 1-6y.o.:* 4mg QD taken in the evening. *Child 6-14y.o.:* 5mg QD taken in the evening. *Adult:* 10mg QD taken in the evening.	B
Moricizine *(Ethmozine)*	*Tab:* 200, 250, 300mg	**Ventricular arrhythmia:** *Adult:* 200-300mg Q 8h.	B
Morphine sulfate *(Roxanol, MS Contin, Oramorph SR, OMS Concentrate, MSIR, RMS)*	*Tab:* Morphine sulfate: 10, 15, 30mg; MSIR: 15mg *Tab (SR):* MS Contin: 15, 30, 60, 100mg; Oramorph SR: 30, 60, 100mg *Liquid:* Morphine sulfate oral sltn, morphine sulfate MSIR: 10, 20mg/5ml; Rescudose: 4 mg/ml; Roxanol conc. oral sltn, MSIR oral sltn concentrate, OMS concentrate, Roxanol 100 concentrated oral solution: 20 mg/ml	**PO:** *Adult (tab, liquid):* 5-30mg Q 4h. *Adult (Tab SR):* 30-100mg or more as needed BID. **PR:** *Adult:* 10-20mg Q 4h prn. **SC/IM/IV:** *Child:* 0.1-0.2mg/kg (max 15mg) Q 2-4h prn. *Adult:* 5-20mg Q 4h prn.	C,D*

See index for proprietary names of generic meds

	Supp: Morphine sulfate suppositories, RMS, or Roxanol: 5, 10, 20, 30mg *Inj:* 0.5, 1, 2, 4, 5, 8, 10, 15, 25mg/ml		
Moricizine **(Ethmozine)**	*Tab:* 200, 250, 300mg *Tab:* 400mg	*Ventricular arrhythmia: Adult:* 200-300mg Q 8h.	C
Moxifloxacin **(Avelox)**	*Inj:* 400mg	*Adult:* 400mg po/IV QD. **Bronchitis**: 5d. **Sinusitis/community-acquired pneumonia:** 10d.	C,D3
Nabumetone **(Relafen)**	*Tab:* 500, 750mg	*Adult:* start 1000mg single dose. Increase to 1500-2000mg/d as single dose or divided BID.	C,D3
Nadolol **(Corgard)**	*Tab:* 20, 40, 80, 120, 160mg	*HTN: Adult:* 40-320mg QD. *Angina: Adult:* 40-240mg QD.	C,D2-3
Nafcillin **(Unipen, Nafcil)**	*Inj:* 0.5, 1.0, 2.0g	*Child ≤7d, <2kg:* 25mg/kg IM/IV Q 12h. *Child ≤7d, >2kg:* 25mg/kg IM/IV Q 8h. *Child >7d-1y.o., <1.2 kg:* 25mg/kg IM/IV Q 12h. *Child >7d-1y.o., 1.2-2kg:* 25mg/kg IM/IV Q 8h. *Child >7d-1y.o., >2kg:* 25mg/kg IM/IV Q 6h. *Child >1y.o.:* **Mild to moderate infection:** 12.5-25mg/kg IM/IV Q 6h. **Severe infection:** 25-50mg/kg (max 3g) IM/IV Q 6h. *Adult:* 500mg IM Q 4-6h or 500-2000mg IV Q 4h.	B
Nalbuphine **(Nubain)**	*Inj:* 10, 20mg/ml	**SC/IM/IV:** *Adult:* 10mg Q 3-6h, max single dose 20mg, max daily dose 160mg.	B

Medication	Preparation	Dosing	Pregnancy Risk
Nalidixic acid *(NegGram)*	*Liquid:* 250mg/5ml *Tab:* 250, 500, 1000mg	*Adult:* 1g Q 6h.	C
Nalmefene *(Revex)*	*Blue label:* 100µg in 1ml (use for post-operative opioid reversal) *Green label:* 2mg in 2ml (use to reverse opioid overdose)	**Postoperative opioid depression** *(Blue label):* *Adult:* 0.25µg/kg IV, then 0.25µg/kg Q 2-5min as needed. Most pts reach max response at dose of 1µg/kg. **Suspected or known opioid overdose** *(Green label):* *Adult:* 0.5mg/70kg IV; if no effect in 2-5min, give 1mg/70kg. Most pts reach max response at dose of 1.5mg/70kg. *Test for opiate withdrawal with 0.1mg/70kg.*	B
Naloxone *(Narcan)*	*Inj:* 0.4, 1mg/ml	**Narcotic overdose: IV/IM:** *Child <20kg:* 0.1mg/kg. *Child >20kg-adult:* 0.4-2mg. May repeat initial dose Q 2-3min prn. *After desired effect obtained, may need to repeat doses Q 20-60min or start infusion at rate/hour = to* $^2/_3$ *of dose at which original response obtained.*	B

Naphazoline ophthalmic *(Allerest, Clear Eyes, Naphcon, Naphcon Forte [0.1%])*	*Sltn:* 0.012% and 0.1% in 15 and 30ml	*Adult:* 1-2 drops Q 3-4h (max 4 times/d).	C
Naproxen *(Naprosyn)*	*Liquid:* 125mg/5ml *Tab:* 220, 250, 375, 500mg	*Child > 2y.o.:* 2.5-10mg/kg BID, max 10mg/kg/d. *Adult:* 250-500mg BID. **Dysmenorrhea:** 500mg, then 250mg Q 6-8h, max 1250mg/d.	B,D3
Naratriptan *(Amerge)*	*Tabs:* 1, 2.5mg	**Migraine headache:** *Adult:* 1-2.5mg, may repeat in 4h, max 5mg/d.	C
Natamycin ophthalmic *(Natacyn)*	*Sltn:* 5% in 15ml	**Antifungal:** *Adult:* 1 drop Q 1-2h for 3-4d, then reduce to 1 drop Q 3-4h, continue treatment for 14-21d.	C
Nedocromil *(Tilade)*	*Inhaler:* 1.75mg/ activation	**Asthma prevention:** *Child >12y.o.-adult:* 2 puffs QID. May reduce to BID-TID once response occurs.	B
Nefazodone *(Serzone)*	*Tab:* 50, 100, 150, 200, 250mg	*Adult <65y.o.:* 200mg/d divided BID. Increase Q 1-2wk by 100-200mg/d until response achieved in range of 300-600mg/d. *Adult >65y.o.:* starting dose is 100mg BID.	C
Nelfinavir *(Viracept)*	*Powder:* 50mg drug/g *Tab:* 250,625mg	*Child 2-13y.o.:* 20-30mg/kg (max 750mg) TID with food. *Adult:* 750mg TID with food.	B

Medication	Preparation	Dosing	Pregnancy Risk
Neomycin	*Liquid:* 125mg/5ml *Tab:* 500mg	***E. coli diarrhea:*** *Child/adult:* 12.5mg/kg Q 6h for 2-3d. ***Hepatic coma:*** *Child:* 50-100mg/kg/d divided Q 6-8h or 2.5-7g/m²/d divided Q 4-6h for 5-6d, max 12g/d. *Adult:* 4-12g/d divided Q 4-6h for max of 2wk. ***Chronic hepatic insufficiency:*** 4g/d divided Q 6-8h for an indefinite period.	C
Neomycin/ polymyxin B/ gramicidin ophthalmic *(Neosporin Ophthalmic Solution, AK-Spore)*	*Sltn:* Neo 1.75mg/Poly 10,000 U/Gram 0.025mg per ml	*Adult:* 1-2 drops into affected eye Q 4h for 7-10d.	NR
Neomycin/ polymyxin B/ hydrocortisone otic *(Cortisporin Otic)*	*Susp:* Neo 3.5mg/Poly 10,000U/Hydro 10mg per ml	*Child/adult:* 3 drops *(child)* or 4 drops *(adult)* in ear TID-QID.	C

See index for proprietary names of generic meds

Neostigmine (*Prostigmin*)	*Inj:* 0.25, 0.5, 1.0mg/ml	***Reversal of non-depolarizing paralyzing agents:*** *Child:* 0.025-0.1mg/kg IV. *Adult:* 0.5-2mg IV, may repeat up to 5mg total IV. *Also give atropine or glycopyrrolate.* ***For emergency treatment of myasthenia:*** see p. 123.	C
Nesiritide (*Natrecor*)	*Inj:* 1.5mg powder	*Adult:* 2μg/kg IV bolus, then 0.01μg/kg/min; titrate with 1μg/kg IV bolus and increase by 0.005μg/kg/min no sooner than 3h to max of 0.03μg/kg/min.	C
Nevirapine (*Viramune*)	*Tab:* 200mg	*Child <2mo.:* 5mg/kg QD for 14d, then 7mg/kg BID. *Child 2mo.-8y.o.:* 4mg/kg QD for 14d, then 7mg/kg BID. *Child >8y.o.:* 4mg/kg QD for 14d, then 4mg/kg BID. *Max child dose is 400mg/d.* *Adult:* 200mg QD for 14d, then 200mg BID.	C

Medication	Preparation	Dosing	Pregnancy Risk
Nicardipine *(Cardene)*	*Cap:* 20, 30mg *Cap (SR):* 30, 45, 60mg *Inj:* 2.5mg/ml	**PO:** *Adult:* 60-120mg/d. Divide TID (cap) or BID (SR). **IV:** *Adult:* start infusion at 5mg/h, increase rate by 2.5mg/h every 5-15min up to max 15mg/h. Decrease to 3mg/h when desired BP obtained.	C
Nicotine *(Commit, Habitrol, Nicoderm, Nicorette, Nicotrol, ProStep)*	*Gum (OTC):* Nicorette: 2, 4mg *Lozenge (OTC):* Commit: 2, 4mg *Inhltn system:* Nicotrol: 10mg cartridge delivers 4mg *Patch:* Nicoderm (OTC): 7, 14, 21mg/d; ProStep: 11, 22mg/d; Nicotrol: 15mg/16h *Nasal spray:* Nicotrol: 0.5mg/spray	**Gum:** 1 piece prn for urge, usual 10-12/d, max 30/d. **Lozenge:** Use 4mg if pt smokes within 30min of waking, otherwise 2mg. *Wk 1-6:* 1 Q 1-2h. *Wk 7-9:* 1 Q 2-4h. *Wk 10-12:* 1 Q 4-8h. **Inhltn system:** frequent continuous puffing for 20min using 6-16 cartridges/d for 3mo., then wean over 6-12wk. **Patch:** Apply patch to clean, non-hairy part of trunk or upper, outer arm. Nicoderm: *<100lb or <10 cigarets/d or CV disease:* One 14mg patch for 6wk, then one 7mg patch for 2wk. *All others:* One 21mg patch QD for 6wk, then one 14mg patch for 2-4wk, then one 7mg patch for 2-4wk. ProStep: *<15 cigarets/d:* One 11mg patch QD for 6wk. *All others:* One 22mg patch QD for 6wk. Nicotrol: One 15mg patch QD for 16 h/d, remove for 8 h/d, for 6wk. Nasal spray: 1-2 sprays/h.	D

Nifedipine (*Procardia, Procardia XL, Adalat*)	*Cap:* 10, 20mg *Tab (XL):* 30, 60, 90mg	*Adult:* Tab <u>XL</u>: 30-120mg QD.	C
Nimodipine (*Nimotop*)	*Cap:* 30mg	***Subarachnoid hemorrhage:*** *Adult:* 60mg Q 4h for 21d.	C
Nisoldipine (*Sular*)	*Tab:* 10, 20, 30, 40mg	*Adult <65y.o.:* start 20mg QD, increase by 10mg/wk as needed, max 60mg/d. *Adult >65y.o.:* start at 10mg/d.	C
Nitazoxanide (*Alinia*)	*Liquid:* 100mg/5ml	*Child 12-47mo.:* 100mg Q 12h × 3d. *Child 4-11y.o.:* 200mg Q 12h × 3d. *Adult:* 500mg QD (not FDA approved).	B
Nitrofurantoin (*Macrodantin, Macrobid*)	*Liquid:* 25mg/5ml *Cap:* 25, 50, 100mg *Cap (SR)* Macrobid: 100mg	*Take all doses with food.* ***UTI treatment:*** *Child >1mo.:* 1.25-1.75mg/kg QID, max 400mg/d. *Adult:* 50-100mg QID. *Cap SR:* 100mg Q 12h. ***UTI prophylaxis:*** *Child >1mo.:* 1mg/kg hs. *Adult:* 50-100mg hs.	B
Nitroglycerin <u>SL tab</u> - *Nitrostat Tab/cap* - *Nitro-Bid, Nitro-Time, Nitroglyn, Nitrong*	*Subling tab:* 0.3, 0.4, 0.6mg *Tab:* 6.5, 9mg *Cap:* 2.5, 6.5, 9, 13mg *Buccal tab:* 2, 3mg	**Subling tab:** 0.15-0.6mg prn for chest pain or expectation of chest pain Q 5min until relief, max 3 doses. **Tab/cap:** 7.5-27mg/d divided Q 8-12h. **Buccal tab:** 1 tab Q 3-5h. Place tab between lip and gum above incisors or between cheek and gum.	B

(continued on following page)

Medication	Preparation	Dosing	Pregnancy Risk
(continued) Nitroglycerin *(continued)* **Buccal (transmucosal) tab** - Nitrogard **Lingual Spray** - Nitrolingual **Transdermal** - Minitran, Deponit, Transderm-Nitro, Nitrodisc, Nitro-Dur, NTS, Nitrek **Ointment** - Nitro-Bid, Nitrol)	*Transdermal patch:* 0.1, 0.2, 0.3, 0.4, 0.6, 0.8mg/h *Lingual spray:* 0.4mg/spray *Topical ointment:* 2% *Inj:* 0.5, 0.8, 5mg/ml	**Transdermal:** 0.1-0.6mg/h patch on for 12-14h/d and off for 10-12h/d. Generally off while sleeping. **Lingual spray:** 1-2 sprays prn for chest pain or expectation of chest pain Q 5min until relief, max 3 doses. **Ointment:** 0.5-5.0inches to skin Q 8h. **IV:** start 10-20µg/min infusion with stepwise increases of 10µg/min Q 3-5min as needed, max 200µg/min.	
Nitroprusside *(Nipride)*	*Inj:* 50mg vial	*Child/adult:* start at 0.5µg/kg/min IV, titrate to max 10µg/kg/min infusion.	C
Nizatidine *(Axid)*	*Cap:* 75 (OTC), 150, 300mg	**Active PUD:** *Adult:* 150mg BID or 300mg hs. **Maintenance PUD:** 150mg hs. **GERD:** 150mg BID.	B
Norepinephrine *(Levophed)*	*Inj:* 1mg/ml	*Child:* initial 0.05-0.1µg/kg/min, max 6µg/kg/min. *Adult:* initial 8-12µg/min. Titrate to response.	C

See index for proprietary names of generic meds

Norfloxacin (*Noroxin*)	*Tab:* 400mg	***UTI:*** *Adult:* 400mg Q 12h for 3-21d. ***GC:*** 800mg po once.	C
Norfloxacin ophthalmic (*Chibroxin*)	*Sltn:* 3mg/ml in 5ml	*Child >1y.o.-adult:* 1-2 drops in affected eye QID for up to 7d. In severe infections, 1-2 drops Q 2h on day 1 only.	NR
Nortriptyline (*Pamelor*)	*Liquid:* 10mg/5ml *Cap:* 10, 25, 50, 75mg	*Adult:* 10-100mg QD or in divided doses.	D
Nystatin (*Mycostatin*)	*Vag tab:* 100,000U *Cream/ointment:* 100,000U/g *Oral susp:* 100,000U/ml *Tab:* 500,000U *Troche:* 200,000U	***Vaginal Candida:*** 1 vag tab hs or 1g cream BID for 14d. ***Cutaneous/mucocutaneous candidiasis:*** apply cream or ointment BID until lesions are healed. ***Thrush/candidal esophagitis:*** **Oral susp:** *Child <1y.o.:* 2ml po QID. *Child >1y.o.- adult:* 4-6ml po QID. Hold in mouth several min before swallowing. HIV pts may use vag tab to prolong contact with mucosa. *Troche: Child/adult:* 1-2 dissolved in mouth 4-5 times/d. ***Intestinal candidiasis:*** 500,000-1,000,000U po TID.	C

Medication	Preparation	Dosing	Pregnancy Risk
Octreotide (*Sandostatin*)	*Inj:* 0.05, 0.1, 0.2mg/ml Depot *inj:* 10, 20, 30mg	***Bleeding esophageal varices:*** *Adult:* 25-50µg IV, then 25-50µg/h infusion. ***Hypoglycemia related to sulfonylurea use:*** *Adult:* 50-75µg IM/IV Q 6h. ***Intractable diarrhea:*** *Child >1y.o.:* 1-10µg/kg/d QD or divided Q 12h SC/IV. May increase by 0.3µg/kg/dose Q 3d to max 10µg/kg/d. *Adult:* 50-100µg IV Q 8h, may increase by 100µg dose Q 2d, max 1500 µg/d.	B
Ofloxacin (*Floxin*)	*Tab:* 200, 300, 400mg *Inj:* 200, 400mg/vial	**PO:** *Adult >18y.o.:* ***Gonorrhea:*** 400mg single dose. ***Chlamydia:*** 300mg Q 12h for 7d. ***UTI:*** 200mg Q 12h for 3d, 7d, or 10d, based on severity. ***Prostatitis:*** 300mg Q 12h for 6wk. ***Respiratory:*** 400mg Q 12h for 10d. ***Skin:*** 400mg Q 12h for 10d. **IV:** *Adult >18y.o.:* ***Respiratory:*** 400mg Q 12h for 10d. ***UTI:*** 200mg Q 12h for 3-10d. ***Skin:*** 400mg Q 12h for 10d.	C
Ofloxacin ophthalmic (*Ocuflox*)	*Sltn:* 3mg/ml in 1 and 5ml	***Conjunctivitis:*** *Adult:* 1-2 drops Q 2-4h for 2d, then 1-2 drops 4 times/d for 5d. ***Corneal ulcer:*** *Adult:* 1-2 drops Q 30 min while awake for 2d, then 1-2 drops Q 1h while awake for 7d, then 1-2 drops QID.	C

See index for proprietary names of generic meds

Ofloxacin otic (Floxin Otic)	*Sltn:* 3mg/ml	**Otitis externa:** *Child 1-10y.o.:* 5 drops BID for 10d. *Child 10y.o.-adult:* 10 drops BID for 10d. **OM with perf. TM:** *Child >12y.o.-adult:* 10 drops BID for 14d.	C
Olanzapine (Zyprexa)	*Tab:* 2.5, 5, 7.5, 10, 15, 20mg	*Adult >18y.o.:* 5-20mg QD.	C
Olmesartan (Benicar)	*Tab:* 5, 20, 40mg	*Adult:* 20mg QD; may titrate up to 40mg QD after 2wk of therapy.	D
Olopatadine ophthalmic (Patanol)	*Sltn:* 0.1% in 5ml	*Child >3y.o.-adult:* 1-2 drops BID.	C
Omeprazole (Prilosec)	*Liquid:* 2mg/ml *Cap:* 10, 20, 40mg	*Child:* 1mg/kg/dose QD-BID *Adult:* **GERD, duodenal ulcer:** 20mg QD. **Gastric ulcer:** 40mg QD.	C
Ondansetron (Zofran)	*Liquid:* 4mg/5ml *Tab:* 4, 8mg Orally disintegrating tab (ODT): 4, 8mg *Inj:* 2mg/ml	**PO:** *Child 4-12y.o.:* 4mg Q 4h for 3 doses, then 4mg Q 8h. *Child >12y.o.-adult:* 8mg Q 4h for 3 doses, then 8mg Q 8h. **IV:** *Child >3y.o.-adult:* 0.15mg/kg. Give first dose 30min before chemotherapy, further doses 4h and 8h later. *Optional dosing: adult (only):* 32mg 30min before chemoRx.	B

Medication	Preparation	Dosing	Pregnancy Risk
Orphenadrine (*Norflex*)	*Tab:* 100mg *Inj:* 30mg/ml	*Adult:* 100mg po BID or 60mg IM/IV Q 12h.	C
Orphenadrine/ aspirin/caffeine (*Norgesic, Norgesic Forte*)	*Tab: Norgesic:* Orph 25mg/ASA 385mg/ Caff 30mg *Tab: Norgesic Forte:* Orph 50mg/ASA 770mg/Caff 60mg	*Adult: Norgesic* 1-2 tabs Q 6-8h. *Norgesic Forte:* 0.5-1 tab Q 6-8h.	C
Oseltamivir (*Tamiflu*)	*Liquid:* 12mg/ml *Cap:* 75mg	**Influenza treatment:** *Child <15kg:* 2mg/kg (max 30mg) BID. *Child 15-23kg:* 45mg BID. *Child 23-40kg:* 60mg BID. *Child >40kg-adult:* 75mg BID. Treat all for 5d. **Influenza prophylaxis:** *Child >12y.o.-adult:* 75mg QD for 7d-6wks.	C
Oxacillin (*Bactocill, Prostaphlin*)	*Inj:* 1, 2, 10g	**IM/IV:** *Child:* 37.5mg/kg Q 6h. *Adult:* 250mg-2g Q 4-6h.	B
Oxaprozin (*Daypro*)	*Tab:* 600mg	*Adult:* 600-1200mg QD.	C,D3
Oxazepam (*Serax*)	*Cap:* 10, 15, 30mg *Tab:* 15mg	*Adult:* **Anxiety:** 10-30mg TID-QID. **Hypnotic:** 15-30mg hs. *Alc. withdrawal:* 15-30mg TID-QID	D

See index for proprietary names of generic meds

Oxcarbazepine *(Trileptal)*	*Liquid:* 300mg/5ml *Tab:* 150, 300, 600mg	*Child 4-16y.o.:* Start 4-5mg/kg, max 300mg, po BID. May increase over 2wk to maintenance BID for *20-29kg:* 450mg/dose; *29-39kg:* 600mg/dose; *>39kg:* 900mg/dose. *Adult:* start 300mg po BID. Increase *if monotherapy:* by 150mg/dose Q 3d to max 600mg po BID; *if adding to other anticonvulsants:* by 300mg/dose Q wk to max 2400mg/d.	C
Oxybutynin *(Ditropan, Ditropan XL, Oxytrol)*	*Liquid:* 5mg/5ml *Tab:* 5mg *Tab XL:* 5, 10mg *Patch:* 36mg	*Child >5y.o.:* 5mg BID-TID. *Adult:* 5mg BID-QID. *Tab XL:* 5-30mg QD. **Patch (Oxytrol):** apply Q 3-4d.	B
Oxycodone *(Roxicodone, OxyFast, OxyContin, OxyIr)*	*Liquid:* 5mg/5ml; 20mg/ml *Cap:* 5mg *Tab:* 5, 10, 15, 20, 30mg *Tab CR:* 10, 20, 40, 80mg *Supp:* 10, 20mg	**PO:** *Child:* 0.05-0.15mg/kg (max 5mg) Q 4-6h. *Adult:* 5-30mg Q 3-6h. *Tab CR:* 10mg Q 12h, increase as needed. **PR:** *Adult:* 10-40mg TID-QID.	B,D*
Oxycodone/acetaminophen *(Tylox, Percocet, Roxilox, Roxicet)*	*Liquid:* Oxy 5mg/Acet 325mg per 5ml *Cap:* Oxy 5mg/Acet 325mg; Oxy 5 mg/Acet 500mg	*Adult:* 1 tab, 1 cap, or 5ml Q 6h prn.	C

(continued on following page)

Medication	Preparation	Dosing	Pregnancy Risk
Oxycodone/aceta-minophen (continued)	*Tab:* Oxy 5mg/Acet 325mg; Oxy 5mg/Acet 500mg; Oxy 7.5mg/Acet 325mg; Oxy 10mg/Acet 325mg		
Oxycodone/aspirin (*Percodan, Rox-iprin, Codoxy*)	*Tab:* Oxy 4.88mg/ASA 325mg	*Adult:* 1-2 tabs Q 6h prn.	D
Oxymetazoline (*Afrin*)	*Drops:* 0.025%, 0.05% *Spray:* 0.05%	*Child 2-5y.o.:* instill 2-3 drops (0.025% sltn) each nostril BID for up to 3d. *Child >6y.o.-adult:* instill 2-3 drops/sprays (0.05% sltn) in each nostril BID. *Do not prescribe for more than 3-5d.*	C
Oxymetazoline ophthalmic (*OcuClear, Visine L.R.*)	*Sltn:* 0.025% in 15 and 30ml	*Child >6y.o.-adult:* 1-2 drops Q 6h.	C
Oxytocin (*Pitocin*)	*Inj:* 10U/ml	***Postpartum bleeding:*** **IM:** 3-10U after delivery. **IV infusion:** 10-40U in 1 liter; infuse at rate needed.	NR
Palonosetron (*Aloxi*)	*Inj:* 0.25mg	*Adult:* 0.25mg IV 30min before chemotherapy.	B

See index for proprietary names of generic meds

Pamidronate *(Aredia)*	*Inj:* 30, 60, 90mg	***Hypercalcemia of malignancy:*** *Ca⁺⁺ 12-13mg/dl:* 60-90mg IV over 2-24h. *Ca⁺⁺ >13.5mg/dl:* 90mg IV over 2-24h. *Wait 7d before re-treating.* ***Paget's disease:*** 30mg in 500ml over 4h IV QD for 3d.	D
Pancuronium *(Pavulon)*	*Inj:* 1, 2mg/ml	***Defasciculating/priming:*** *Child/adult:* 0.01mg/kg IV. ***Acute paralyzing dose:*** *Child <1mo.:* 0.02mg/kg IV. *Child >1mo.-adult:* 0.04-0.1mg/kg IV. ***Intermittent:*** *Child <1mo.:* 0.03-0.09mg/kg Q 1-3h. *Child >1mo.-adult:* 0.1mg/kg Q 1-3h. ***Infusion:*** *Child >1mo.-adult:* 0.06-0.1mg/kg/h.	C
Pantoprazole *(Protonix)*	*Tab:* 40mg *Inj:* 40mg/vial	*Adult:* **PO/IV:** *GERD:* 40mg QD. *PUD:* 40-80mg QD. **Hypersecretory conditions:** 40-120mg <u>BID</u>.	B
Papaverine *(Pavabid)*	*Cap:* 150mg *Inj:* 30mg/ml	*Adult:* **PO:** start 150mg Q 12h. May increase to 150mg Q 8h or 300mg Q 12h. **IV:** 30-120mg Q 3h.	C
Paroxetine *(Paxil)*	*Liquid:* 10mg/5ml *Tab:* 10, 20, 30, 40mg *Tab CR:* 12.5, 25mg	*Adult:* 20-60mg QD. <u>Tab <u>CR</u>:</u> 12.5-75mg QD.	C

Medication	Preparation	Dosing	Pregnancy Risk
Penciclovir (*Denavir*)	*Cream:* 1%	*Adult:* apply Q 2h to skin for 4d while awake. Begin treatment as soon as possible.	B
Penicillin G	*Inj:* 200,000, 500,000, 1 million, 5 million, 10 million, 20 millionU	*Child <7d:* **Meningitis:** 83,000-150,000U/kg IM/IV Q 8h. *Child 7d-1y.o.:* **Meningitis:** 150,000U/kg IM/IV Q 6h. *Child >1y.o.:* **Meningitis:** 250,000U/kg/d IM/IV divided Q 3-4h. *Child <7d:* **Other:** 17,000U/kg IM/IV Q 8h. *Child >7d:* **Other:** 25,000-50,000U/kg IM/IV Q 8h. *Adult, low dose (LD):* 4-6 millionU/d IV divided Q 4-6h. *Adult, medium dose (MD):* 8-12 millionU/d IV divided Q 4-6h. *Adult, high dose (HD):* 12-30 millionU/d IV divided Q 3-4h.	B
Penicillin V	*Liquid:* 125mg (200,000U), 250mg (400,000U)/5ml *Tab:* 125, 250, 500mg	*Child:* 6-12mg/kg (max 500mg) Q 6h. *Adult:* 250-500mg Q 6-8h.	B
Pentamidine (*NebuPent, Pentam 300*)	*Sltn for inhalation:* 300mg *Inj:* 300mg	**Pneumocystis treatment and prophylaxis:** see pp. 129-130.	C

Pentazocine *(Talwin)*	*Tab:* 50mg with naloxone 0.5mg *Inj:* 30mg/ml	**PO:** *Adult:* 50-100mg Q 3-4h, max 600mg/d. **SC/IM:** *Adult:* 30-60mg Q 3-4h, max 360mg/d. **IV:** *Adult:* 30mg Q 3-4h prn.	C,D*
Pentobarbital *(Nembutal)*	*Inj:* 50mg/ml	*Sedation: Child:* 1-3mg/kg IV, max 100mg/d. *Adult:* 100-200mg IV at 50mg/min. Additional doses Q 1-5min to max 500mg total.	D
Pentoxifylline *(Trental)*	*Tab:* 400mg	*Adult:* 400mg TID with meals. Reduce to 400mg BID if GI or CNS symptoms occur.	C
Permethrin *(Elimite, Nix)*	*Cream:* tube 60g of 5% *Crème rinse:* 2fl oz of 1% *Lotion:* 1%	*Lice:* see p. 117. *Scabies:* see p. 133.	B
Perphenazine *(Trilafon)*	*Syrup:* 2mg/5ml *Tab:* 2, 4, 8, 16mg *Concentrate PO:* 16mg/5ml *Inj:* 5mg/ml	*Psychosis:* **PO:** *Adult:* 4-16mg BID-QID, max 64mg/d. **IM:** *Adult:* initial dose 5mg Q 6h, up to 10mg Q 6h, max 15mg/d in ambulatory patients and 30mg/d in inpatients. *Nausea/vomiting:* **PO:** *Adult:* 8-24mg/d divided BID-QID. **IM:** *Adult:* initial dose 5mg Q 6h, up to 10mg Q 6h, max 15mg/d in ambulatory patients and 30mg/d in inpatients. **IV:** *Adult:* 1mg at 1-2min intervals up to a total of 5mg.	C

Medication	Preparation	Dosing	Pregnancy Risk
Phenazopyridine *(Azo-Gesic, AzoStandard, Prodium, Pyridium, Re-Azo, Uristat, UTI Relief)*	*Tab:* 95, 100, 200mg	*Child 6-12y.o.:* 4mg/kg TID for 2d. *Child 12y.o.-adult:* 100-200mg TID for 2d.	B
Phenelzine *(Nardil)*	*Tab:* 15mg	**Initiation:** *Adult:* 15-30mg po TID. *Elderly adult:* 5-20mg po TID.	C
Phenobarbital *(Barbita, Solfoton, Luminal)*	*Liquid:* 15, 20mg/5ml *Tab:* 8, 15, 16, 30, 32, 60, 65, 100mg *Cap:* 16mg *Inj:* 30, 60, 65, 130mg/ml	**IV loading dose:** *Child/adult:* 15-20mg/kg at 30mg/min *(child)* or 60mg/min *(adult).* **PO maintenance:** *Child <1mo.:* 3-5mg/kg QD or div BID. *Child 1mo.-1y.o.:* 5-8mg/kg QD or div BID. *Child 1-5y.o.:* 6-8mg/kg QD or div BID. *Child 6-12y.o.:* 4-6mg/kg QD or div BID. *Child >12y.o.-adult:* 1-3mg/kg QD or div BID.	D
Phenobarbital/ ergotamine/ belladonna *(Bellergal-S)*	*Tab:* Phenobarbital 40mg/Ergotamine 0.6mg/Belladonna 0.2mg	*Adult:* 1 tab BID.	X

See index for proprietary names of generic meds

	Tab/Cap/Liquid per		
Phenobarbital/hyoscyamine/atropine/scopolamine *(Donnatal)*	*5ml:* Phen 16.2mg/ Hyos 0.1037mg/ Atro 0.0194mg/ Scop 0.0065mg	*Child:* 0.1ml/kg Q 4h. *Adult:* 1-2 tab(s) or cap(s) or 5-10ml TID-QID.	D
Phentolamine *(Regitine)*	*Inj:* 5mg/ml	*Adrenergic drug extravasation:* **SC:** *Child:* 0.1-0.2mg/kg (max 10mg). Dilute in 10ml 0.9% NS, infiltrate within 12h. *Adult:* 5-10mg in 10ml 0.9% NS. Infiltrate within 12h. *Hypertensive crisis:* *Adult:* 5-20mg IV.	C
Phenylephrine	*Inj:* 1%	*Hypotension/shock:* **IM/SC:** *Child:* 0.1 mg/kg (max 5mg) Q 1-2h prn. **IV bolus:** 5-20μg/kg Q 10-15min prn. **IV infusion:** 0.1-0.5μg/kg/min. *Adult:* **IM/SC:** 2-5mg Q 1-2h prn. **IV bolus:** 0.1-0.5mg Q 10-15min prn. **IV infusion:** 0.05-0.1mg/min, titrate to maintain BP.	C
Phenylephrine ophthalmic *(Relief, Prefrin Liquifilm, Neo-Synephrine, Mydfrin 2.5%)*	*Sltn:* 0.12% and 2.5% in 2, 5, and 15ml; 10% in 2 and 5ml	*Irritation:* *Adult:* use 1 to 2 drops of 0.12% sltn up to QID. *Dilation and glaucoma:* 2.5% or 10% 1 drop as needed.	C

Medication	Preparation	Dosing	Pregnancy Risk
Phenytoin (*Dilantin*)	*Tab (chew)*: 50mg *Cap*: 30, 100mg *Cap (ER)* 30, 100mg *Susp*: 30, 125mg/5ml *Inj*: 50mg/ml	***PO loading:*** *Adult*: 17-20mg/kg po single dose. *May take 12h or more to reach therapeutic level.* ***IV loading:*** *Child/adult*: 15-18mg/kg at 25-30mg/min, in emergencies max infusion rate 50mg/min. ***Seizure maintenance:*** *Child*: 4-8mg/kg/d divided Q 8-12h. *Adult*: 300-600mg/d (usually 300mg/d) divided Q 8-24h.	D
Phytonadione (Vitamin K1) (***AquaMEPHYTON,*** ***Mephyton***)	*Tab*: 5mg *Inj*: 0.5mg/ml, 10mg/ml	***Oral anticoagulant overdose:*** *Infants*: **SC:** 1-2mg Q 4-8h. *Child/Adult*: **PO/IV/SC:** 2.5-10mg. *May repeat in 6-8h if given IM, IV, SC; in 12-48h if po.* See page 80 for recommendations on therapeutic warfarin OD.	C
Pilocarpine ophthalmic (*Isopto Carpine, Pilocar, Piloptic, Pilostat*)	*Sltn*: 0.25%, 0.5%, 1%, 2%, 3%, 4%, 5% 6% in 15 and 30ml	***Glaucoma (miotic):*** *Adult*: 1 or 2 drops in affected eye TID-QID.	C
Pimecrolimus (*Elidel*)	*Cream*: 1% 15, 30, 100g tube	*Adult*: apply to affected areas BID.	C
Pindolol (*Visken*)	*Tab*: 5, 10mg	*Adult*: 10-60mg/d divided Q 8-12h.	B,D2-3

Pioglitazone *(Actos)*	*Tab:* 15, 30, 45mg	*Adult:* 15-45mg QD.	C
Pipecuronium *(Arduan)*	*Inj:* 10mg	*Child/adult:* initial 70-85µg/kg IV, subsequent doses of 10-15µg/kg IV as needed. *Dose by ideal BW. Children 1-14y.o. may need larger doses.*	C
Piperacillin *(Pipracil)*	*Inj:* 2, 3, 4g	*Child >12y.o.:* **IM/IV:** 200-300mg/kg/d in divided doses Q 4-6h. *Adult:* **IM:** 2-3g Q 6-12h. **IV:** 3-4g Q 4-6h. *Max dose for child/adult: 24g/d.*	B
Piperacillin/ tazobactam *(Zosyn)*	*Inj:* Pip 2g/Taz 0.25g; Pip 3g/Taz 0.375g; Pip 4g/Taz 0.5g	*Child >12y.o.-adult:* Pip 3g/Taz 0.375g Q 6h or Pip 4g/Taz 0.5g IV Q 8h.	B
Pirbuterol *(Maxair)*	*Inhaler:* 200µg/puff	*Child >12y.o.-adult:* 1-2 puffs Q 4-6h.	C
Piroxicam *(Feldene)*	*Tab:* 10, 20mg	*Adult:* 20-40mg/d QD or divided BID. *Elderly start at 10mg QD.*	C,D3
Pneumococcal vaccine *(Pneumovax 23)*	*Inj:* 0.5ml dose	*Child >2y.o.-adult:* **IM/SC:** 0.5ml.	C
Polyethylene glycol *(GoLYTELY)*	*Powder* for oral solution	***Drug OD:*** *Child:* 25ml/kg/h until rectal effluent clear. *Adult:* 240ml every 10min until rectal effluent clear or 4liters have been consumed.	C

Medication	Preparation	Dosing	Pregnancy Risk
Pralidoxime *(Protopam Chloride)*	*Inj:* 1g/vial; 600mg/ auto-injector	***Carbamate OD:*** see p. 58. ***Organophosphate OD:*** see p. 60.	C
Pravastatin *(Pravachol)*	*Tab:* 10, 20, 40, 80mg	*Adult:* start 10-20mg hs. Adjust dosage Q 4wk based on response. Max 80mg/d.	X
Praziquantel *(Biltricide)*	*Tab:* 600mg	***Worms:*** see pp. 143-144.	B
Prazosin *(Minipress)*	*Cap:* 1, 2, 5mg	*Adult:* initial dose 1mg BID to TID, usual maintenance 3-15mg/d in 2-3 divided doses, max 20mg/d.	C
Prednisolone *(Prelone, Pediapred)*	*Liquid:* 5mg/5ml; 15mg/5ml	*Dosage dependent on disease process being treated.*	C,D1
Prednisolone ophthalmic *(Econopred, AK-Pred, pred Forte)*	*Susp:* 0.125% in 5, 10ml; <u>Forte</u>: 1% in 5, 10ml *Sltn:* 0.125% and 1% in 5, 10ml	*Adult:* 1-2 drops BID-QID. *Shake well before use.*	C
Prednisone	*Oral sltn:* 5mg/ml; 5mg/5ml *Syrup:* 5mg/5ml *Tab:* 1, 2.5, 5, 10, 20, 25, 50mg	*Dosage dependent on disease process being treated.*	C,D1

See index for proprietary names of generic meds

Primidone (*Mysoline*)	*Liquid:* 250mg/5ml *Tab:* 50, 250mg Chew tab: 125mg	***Seizure maintenance:*** *Child <8y.o.:* 10-25mg/kg/d divided Q 6-8h. *Child >8y.o.-adult:* 0.75-2g/d divided TID-QID.	D
Probenecid (*Benemid*)	*Tab:* 500mg	***Gout maintenance:*** *Adult:* start 250mg BID for 1wk, then 500mg BID, then adjust dose to max 3 g/d.	C
Procainamide (*Procanbid, Pronestyl, Pronestyl SR*)	*Cap:* 250, 375, 500mg *Inj:* 100mg/ml; 500mg/ml *Tab:* 250, 375, 500mg *Tab (SR):* 250, 500, 750, 1000mg *Tab (Procanbid):* 500, 1000mg	**PO:** *Child:* 15-50mg/kg/d divided Q 3-6h max 4g/d. *Adult:* 250-500mg Q 3-6h. <u>SR:</u> 500-1000mg Q 6h. <u>Procanbid:</u> 500-1000mg Q 12h. Usual dose 50mg/kg/d. *Max dose 4g/d.* **IM:** *Child:* 20-30mg/kg/d divided Q 4-6h. *Adult:* 0.5-1g Q 4-8h. *Max dose 4g/d.* **IV load:** *Child:* 3-6mg/kg (max 100mg) over 5min. Repeat Q 5-10min to max 15mg/kg. *Max per 30min is 500mg. Adult:* 17mg/kg load at rate 20mg/min. **IV infusion:** *Child:* 20-80µg/kg/min, max 2g/d. *Adult:* 1-4 mg/min, max 2g/d.	C
Prochlorperazine (*Compazine*)	*Liquid:* 5mg/5ml *Tab:* 5, 10, 25mg Tab SR: 10, 15, 30mg *Cap (SR):* 10, 15, 30mg *Supp:* 2.5, 5, 25mg *Inj:* 5mg/ml	**PO:** *Child >9kg, >2y.o.:* 0.4mg/kg Q 6h. *Adult:* 5-10mg Q 6h. <u>Tab/cap SR:</u> 10-30mg QD-BID. **PR:** *Child >9kg, >2y.o.:* 0.4mg/kg Q 6h. *Adult:* 25mg Q 12h. **Parenteral:** *Child >9kg and >2y.o.:* 0.13mg/kg IM Q 6h. *Adult:* 5-10mg IM/IV Q 6h, max 40mg/d	C

Medication	Preparation	Dosing	Pregnancy Risk
Promethazine *(Phenergan)*	*Liquid:* 6.25, 25mg/5ml *Tab:* 12.5, 25, 50mg *Supp:* 12.5, 25, 50mg *Inj:* 25, 50mg/ml	**PO/PR/IM/IV:** *Child >2y.o.:* 0.25-1mg/kg (max 25mg) Q 4-6h. *Adult:* 12.5-25mg Q 4-6h.	C
Propafenone *(Rythmol)*	*Tab:* 150, 225, 300mg	***Ventricular arrhythmias:*** *Adult:* 150mg Q 8h, increase at 3-4d intervals, max 300mg Q 8h.	C
Proparacaine ophthalmic *(Alcaine, Ophthetic, Ophthaine)*	*Sltn:* 0.5% in 2 and 15ml	*Adult:* 1-2 drops. Not for prolonged use.	C
Propofol *(Diprivan)*	*Inj:* 10mg/ml	***Conscious sedation for procedures:*** *Healthy adult <55y.o.:* 0.5mg/kg IV over 3-5min, then infusion at 25-75µg/kg/min or further boluses of 10-20mg as needed. *Adult >55y.o., debilitated, hypovolemic, or unstable:* give normal loading dose IV over 5min, then 20-60µg/kg/min infusion. *No bolus dosing* ***Sedation of intubated patients:*** *Adult:* initial 5µg/kg/min IV for 5min, then as needed further doses of 5-10µg/kg/min over 5-10min. Maintenance infusion is 5-50µg/kg/min.	B

See index for proprietary names of generic meds

Propoxyphene *(Darvon)*	*Tab:* 65mg	*Adult:* 1 tab Q 4h prn.	C,D*
Propoxyphene/ acetaminophen *(Darvocet-N 50 and 100, Wygesic)*	*Tab:* Darvocet-N 50: Prop 50/Acet 325mg; Darvocet-N 100: Prop 100/Acet 650mg; Wygesic: Prop 65/ Acet 650mg	*Adult:* Darvocet-N 100/Wygesic: 1 tab Q 4h prn. Darvocet-N 50: 2 tabs Q 4h prn.	NR
Propranolol *(Inderal)*	*Liquid:* 20, 40mg/5ml; 80mg/ml *Tab:* 10, 20, 40, 60, 80, 90mg *Cap (SR):* 60, 80, 120, 160mg *Inj:* 1mg/ml	**PO:** *Child:* 0.5-4mg/kg/d divided BID-QID. *Adult:* **HTN:** start 40mg BID. Usual maint. 120-240mg/d divided BID-TID, max 640mg/d. *Cap SR:* 80-160mg QD. **Angina:** 80-320mg/d div BID-QID. **Migraine:** 80-240mg/d div BID-QID. **IV:** *Child:* 0.01-0.1mg/kg (*max* <1y.o.: 1mg; *max* >1y.o.: 3mg) over 10min Q 6-8h prn. *Adult:* 1-3mg Q 5min to desired effect (max total 5mg).	C,D2-3
Propylthiouracil *(PTU)*	*Tab:* 50mg	*Child 6-10y.o.:* start 50-150mg/d divided Q 8h. *Child >10y.o.:* start 150-300mg/d divided Q 8h. *Maintenance dose determined by response, generally begins after 2mo, and is usually* $^1/_3$-$^2/_3$ *of initial dose.* *Adult:* usual starting dose 300-450mg/d (but some may require up to 600-1200mg/d), divided Q 8h. *Usual maintenance 100-150mg/d, max 600-900mg/d.*	D

Medication	Preparation	Dosing	Pregnancy Risk
Prostaglandin E₁	Inj: 500µg/ml	Child <1mo.: start 0.05-0.1µg/kg/min IV, advance to 0.4µg/kg/min IV as needed. When paO₂ increases, decrease to lowest effective dose. Monitor respirations.	NR
Protamine sulfate	Inj: 10mg/ml	Child/adult: 1mg for each 100U heparin to be reversed over 10min IV, max 50mg over any 10min.	C
Prussian blue (Radiogardase)	Cap: 500mg	Child 2-12y.o.: 1g TID. Adult: 3g TID (may be reduced after initial treatment to 1-2g TID).	C
Pseudoephedrine (Sudafed)	Liquid: 7.5mg/0.8ml; 15, 30mg/5ml Tab: 30, 60mg Tab SR: 120, 240mg Cap: 60mg Cap SR: 120mg	Child 2-5y.o.: 15mg Q 6h, max 60mg/d. Child 6-11y.o.: 30mg Q 6h, max 120mg/d. Adult: 30-60mg Q 4-6h or 120mg SR Q 12h, max 240mg/d.	C
Pyrantel pamoate (Antiminth, Pin-X, Pin-Rid)	Liquid: 50mg/ml Cap: 180mg	Worms: see pp. 143-144.	C
Pyrazinamide	Tab: 500mg	TB: Child: 15-30mg/kg/d QD, max 2g/d. Adult: 25mg/kg QD, max 2.5g/d.	C

Pyrethrins with piperonyl butox-ide *(RID)*	*Liquid:* 59, 120, 177, 237ml *Shampoo:* 2, 4, 8fl oz *Gel:* 30g	*Lice:* see p. 117.	C
Pyrimethamine *(Daraprim)*	*Tab:* 25mg	***Toxoplasmosis:*** see p. 138. Pyrimethamine with sulfadoxine: see p. 264.	C
Quetiapine *(Seroquel)*	*Tab:* 25, 100, 200mg	*Adult:* start 25mg BID, usual dose range 75-375mg BID.	C
Quinapril *(Accupril)*	*Tab:* 5, 10, 20, 40mg	*Adult:* 5-80mg/d QD or divided BID.	C,D2-3
Quinidine gluconate *(Quinaglute)*	*Tab SR:* 324mg *Inj:* 80mg/ml	**PO:** *Adult:* 324-648mg Q 8-12h. **IM:** *Adult:* start 400mg, then 400mg Q 4-6h. *If emergency:* 400mg Q 2h, max 5 doses. **IV:** *Adult:* **Arrhythmia:** 800mg in 50cc D_5W at 10mg/min; stop if QRS widens, HR <120bpm, or sinus rhythm resumes. **Malaria:** see pp. 119-120.	C
Quinidine polygalac-turonate *(Cardioquin)*	*Tab:* 275mg (equiva-lent to 200mg of sulfate)	***To terminate arrhythmias:*** *Adult:* start 1-3 tabs Q 3-4h for 3-4 doses. If no effect, increase dose by $\frac{1}{2}$-1 tab and repeat Q 3-4h for 3-4 doses. *Maintenance:* *Adult:* 1 tab BID-TID.	C

Medication	Preparation	Dosing	Pregnancy Risk
Quinidine sulfate (*Quinidex*)	*Tab:* 200, 300mg *Tab* (Quinidex Extentab): 300mg	**PO:** *Child:* **Maintenance:** usual 6mg/kg (range 3.75-15mg/kg) Q 6h. *Adult:* **To terminate arrhythmias:** 200-600mg Q 1-4h until desired effect. **Maintenance:** 200-300mg TID-QID or Quinidex Extentabs: 300-600mg Q 8-12h.	C
Quinine	*Tab:* 260mg *Cap:* 200, 260, 325mg	*Malaria:* see pp. 119-120.	X
Quinupristin/ dalfopristin (*Synercid*)	*Inj:* Quin 150mg/Dalf 350mg	*Adult:* **Vancomycin-resistant enterococcus:** 7.5mg/kg IV Q 8h. **Skin/soft tissue infection:** 7.5mg/kg Q 12h.	B
Rabeprazole (*Aciphex*)	*Tab:* 20mg	*Adult:* **Acute duodenal ulcer:** 20mg QD for up to 4wk. **GERD:** 20mg QD. **Hypersecretory conditions, including Z-E syndrome:** usual 60mg QD, up to 60mg BID for up to 1yr.	B
Rabies immune globulin	*Inj:* 150IU/ml	**Rabies prophylaxis:** see pp. 43 and 133 and rabies vaccine below.	C
Rabies vaccine	*Inj:* Human diploid cell (HDCV) and rabies adsorbed (RVA): 2.5IU/vial	**Rabies prophylaxis:** see pp. 43 and 133 and rabies immune globulin above.	C
Raloxifene (*Evista*)	*Tab:* 60mg	*Osteoporosis: Adult:* 60mg QD.	X

See index for proprietary names of generic meds

Ramipril *(Altace)*	*Cap:* 1.25, 2.5, 5, 10mg	*Adult:* 1.25-20mg/d QD or divided BID.	C,D2-3
Ranitidine *(Zantac)*	*Syrup:* 15mg/ml *Cap (GELdose):* 150, 300mg *Tab:* 75 (OTC), 150, 300mg *Tab (EFFERdose):* 150mg *Granules (EFFERdose):* 150mg *Inj:* 25mg/ml	*Child:* **PO:** *Active PUD/gastritis:* 1-2mg/kg, max 150mg, BID. *Maintenance PUD/gastritis:* 1-2mg/kg, max 75mg, BID. *GERD:* 2.5-5mg BID, max 150mg/dose, unless erosive esophagitis, in which case max 300 mg/dose. **IV:** *PUD/GERD:* 2-4 mg/kg/d divided Q 6-8h, max 150mg/d. *Adult:* **Short-term treatment of PUD:** 150mg po Q 12h or 300mg po hs. *GERD:* 150mg po Q 12h. *Erosive esophagitis:* 150mg po QID. *Prophylaxis of recurrent duodenal ulcer:* 150mg po hs. *Gastric hypersecretory conditions:* **PO:** 150mg Q 12h up to 6g/d. **IM/IV:** 50mg Q 6-8h. **Continuous IV infusion:** 50mg, then 6.25mg/h, titrate to gastric pH >4 for prophylaxis or >7 for treatment.	B
Remifentanil *(Ultiva)*	*Inj:* 1, 2, 5mg	*Conscious sedation for procedures: Child >2y.o.-adult:* **Single IV dose method:** 0.5-1.0μg/kg over 30-60sec. **Continuous infusion method:** start 0.05-0.1μg/kg/ min, adjust by 0.025μg/kg/min Q 5min as needed. *Max infusion rate* 2μg/kg/min. *Reduce dose by 50% in elderly.*	C

Medication	Preparation	Dosing	Pregnancy Risk
Repaglinide (*Prandin*)	*Tab*: 0.5, 1, 2mg	*Adult*: usual dose range 0.5-4mg with meals, max 16mg/d.	C
Reteplase (*Retavase*)	*Powder*: 10.4IU	**Acute MI/PE with hemodynamic compromise:** *Adult*: 10U IV over 2min, repeat dose in 30min.	C
Ribavirin (*Virazole*)	*Inhalation sltn*: 6g/100ml	**Aerosol:** *Child*: dilute 6g in 300ml sterile water for 20mg/ml solution. Administer over 12-18h QD for 3-7d.	X
Rifabutin (*Mycobutin*)	*Cap*: 150mg	**Prevention of disseminated Mycobacterium avium complex in advanced HIV:** 300mg QD. If patient likely to have GI upset, use 150mg BID.	B
Rifampin (*Rifadin*)	*Cap*: 150, 300mg *Inj*: 600mg/vial	**TB:** *Child >5y.o.*: 10-20mg/kg (max 600mg) po/IV QD. *Adult*: 600mg po/IV QD. **Meningitis prophylaxis:** see p. 122.	C
Rimantadine (*Flumadine*)	*Liquid*: 50mg/5ml *Tab*: 100mg	**Influenza A:** *Child <10y.o.*: 5mg/kg (max 150mg) QD. *Child >10y.o.-adult*: 100mg BID; decrease to 100mg/d in elderly or pts with severe hepatic or renal insufficiency. *Treat for 7d after onset of symptoms.*	C
Risperidone (*Risperdal*)	*Liquid*: 1mg/ml *Tab*: 0.25, 0.5, 1, 2, 3, 4mg	*Adult*: start 2mg/d, divided QD-BID, slowly increase to 4-8 mg/d.	C

See index for proprietary names of generic meds

Ritonavir (*Norvir*)	*Liquid*: 80mg/ml *Cap*: 100mg	*Child*: initial 250mg/m^2 BID, titrate to 400mg/m^2 BID, max 600mg/d. *Adult*: start 300mg BID, titrate to 600mg BID with meals.	B
Rizatriptan (*Maxalt, Maxalt-MLT*)	*Tab*: 5, 10mg (disintegrates in mouth)	*Migraine headache*: *Adult*: 5-10mg, may repeat in 2h, max 30mg/d.	C
Rocuronium (*Zemuron*)	*Inj*: 10mg/ml	*Rapid-sequence intubation*: *Child/adult*: 0.6-1mg/kg IV. *Maintenance of paralysis*: **Single IV dose method**: *Child*: 0.075-0.125mg/kg. *Adult*: 0.1-0.2mg/kg. **Continuous infusion method**: *Child/adult*: 0.01-0.012mg/kg/min.	C
Rosiglitazone (*Avandia*)	*Tab*: 2, 4, 8mg	*Adult*: usual starting dose 4mg/d. After 8-12wk, may increase to 8mg/d. Give QD or divided BID.	C
Rosuvastatin (*Crestor*)	*Tab*: 5, 10, 20, 40mg	*Adult*: 5-40mg QD.	C
Salmeterol (*Serevent*)	*Aerosol*: 21μg/puff *Diskus*: 50μg/inhalation	*Aerosol*: *Child >12y.o.-adult*: 2 puffs Q 12h. *Diskus*: *Child >4y.o.-adult*: 1 inhalation BID.	C
Salsalate (*Disalcid*)	*Cap*: 500mg *Tab*: 500, 750mg	*Adult*: 3g/d divided BID-TID.	C

Medication	Preparation	Dosing	Pregnancy Risk
Saquinavir (*Fortovase*, *Invirase*)	*Cap:* 200mg soft gel (Fortovase); 200mg hard gel (Invirase)	*Should be prescribed by brand name. Fortovase has greater bioavailability than Invirase, the older formulation. Adult:* Fortovase 1200mg TID or <u>Invirase</u> 600mg TID with food.	B
Scopolamine (*Transderm Scóp*)	*Transderm patch:* 1.5mg	*Adult:* apply patch behind the ear 4h before time anti-emetic action is required. Duration of action: 72h.	C
Scopolamine ophthalmic (*Isopto Hyoscine*)	*Sltn:* 0.25% in 5 and 15ml	*Uveitis: Adult:* 1-2 drops up to QID.	C
Selegiline (*Eldepryl, Carbex*)	*Cap/tab:* 5mg	*Parkinson's not responding to levodopa/carbidopa: Adult:* 5mg with breakfast and lunch.	C
Selenium sulfide (*Selsun*)	*Lotion/Shampoo:* 1%, 2.5% (120, 210, 240ml bottles)	*Dandruff, seborrheic dermatitis of the scalp:* apply 5-10ml to wet scalp, allow to remain on scalp 2-3min, rinse thoroughly. Repeat and rinse thoroughly. Apply twice each wk for 2wk. Then apply at less frequent intervals: Q 2wk-Q 4wk. *Tinea versicolor:* apply to affected areas and lather with a small amount of water. Allow to remain on skin for 10min, then rinse. Repeat QD for 7d.	NR

See index for proprietary names of generic meds

Sertaconazole (Ertaczo)	*Cream: 2% 15g*	*Adult:* Apply topically to affected area BID.	C
Sertraline (Zoloft)	*Sltn:* 20mg/ml *Tab:* 25, 50, 100mg	*Child 6-12y.o.:* initial dose 25mg QD. Dose may be increased Q wk to a max of 200mg/d. *Child >13y.o.-adult:* initial dose 50mg QD. Dose may be increased Q wk to a max of 200mg/d.	B
Sildenafil citrate (Viagra)	*Tab:* 25, 50, 100mg	*Adult male:* 25-100mg (usually 50mg) 30min-4h (usually 1h) before sexual activity, max QD.	B
Silver sulfadiazine (Silvadene)	*Cream 1%:* 20, 25, 50, 85, 400, 1000g containers	*Child/adult:* Apply 2mm coat QD or BID to affected area.	B
Simethicone (Gas-X, Mylanta Gas, Mylicon, Phazyme)	*Liquid:* 40mg/0.6ml (30ml bottles) *Cap:* 125mg *Tab (chew):* 80, 125mg *Tab (EC):* 60, 95mg	*Sltn: Child <2y.o.:* 20mg QID; max 240mg/d. May mix with infant formula or 30ml of water. *Child 2-12y.o.:* 40mg QID. *Adult:* 40-125mg QID, max 500mg/d. *Take after meals and hs.* *Cap: Adult:* 125mg QID after each meal and hs. *Tab: Adult:* 40-125mg QID after each meal and hs.	C
Simvastatin (Zocor)	*Tab:* 5, 10, 20, 40, 80mg	*Adult:* Usual starting dose 20mg hs, dosage range: 5-80mg/d. Adjust dose at 4wk intervals.	X

Medication	Preparation	Dosing	Pregnancy Risk
Sodium chloride, hypertonic ophthalmic (*Muroptic-5, Muro 128*)	*Sltn:* 2% and 5% in 15ml *Ointment:* 5% in 3.5g	*Adult: Corneal edema:* Sltn: 1-2 drops Q 3-4h. Ointment: $\frac{1}{4}$ inch Q 3-4h.	A
Sodium polystyrene sulfonate (*Kayexalate*)	*Liquid:* 15g/60ml	*Child:* 1g/kg po Q 6h or as retention enema Q 2-6h. *Adult:* 15-60g po or 30-50g in 100ml retention enema Q 6h.	C
Sotalol (*Betapace*)	*Tab:* 80, 120, 160, 240mg	*Adult:* initial dose 80mg BID. Dose may be increased every 2-3d to range of 160-320mg/d, divided BID-TID.	B,D2-3
Sparfloxacin (*Zagam*)	*Tab:* 200mg	*Adult >18y.o.:* 400mg on day 1, then 200mg QD for 9d.	C
Spectinomycin (*Trobicin*)	*Inj:* 2, 4g	*Uncomplicated gonorrhea: Adult:* 2g IM.	B
Spironolactone (*Aldactone*)	*Tab:* 25, 50, 100mg	*Edema: Child:* 1-3mg/kg/d divided BID-QID, max 200mg/d. *Adult:* initial dose 100mg/d, adjust to 25-200mg/d, divide BID-QID. *HTN: Child:* 1-2mg/kg BID. *Adult:* initial 50-100mg/d in single or divided doses, max 400mg/d.	C,D(Htn)

Drug	Formulations	Dosage	Preg
Stavudine (d4t) *(Zerit)*	*Powder for oral solution:* 1mg/1ml *Cap:* 15, 20, 30, 40mg *Cap XR:* 37.5, 50, 75, 100mg	**Powder/cap:** *Child <30kg:* 1mg/kg (max 30mg) BID. *Child 30-60kg, adult<60kg:* 30mg BID. *Adult ≥60kg:* 40mg BID. **Cap XR:** *Adult <60kg:* 75mg QD. *Adult ≥60kg:* 100mg QD. ***Dosage adjustments for renal impairment in adults (use regular tabs/powder):*** *CrCl* *Pt wt ≥60kg* *Pt wt <60kg* *>50 ml/min* 40mg Q 12h 30mg Q 12h *26-50 ml/min* 20mg Q 12h 15mg Q 12h *10-25 ml/min* 20mg Q 24h 15mg Q 24h	C
Streptokinase *(Streptase)*	*Inj:* 250,000U; 750,000U; 1,500,000U	***Myocardial infarction:*** see p. 101-102. ***Venous thrombosis, deep:*** see p. 143. ***Pulmonary embolus:*** see pp. 132-133.	C
Succinylcholine *(Anectine, Quelicin)*	*Inj:* 20, 50, 100mg/ml	***Paralysis for rapid sequence intubation:*** *Child/adult:* 1.0-1.5mg/kg IV. See p. 15 for RSI protocol.	C
Sucralfate *(Carafate)*	*Liquid:* 1g/10ml *Tab:* 1g	***Active duodenal ulcer:*** *Adult:* 1g QID on empty stomach (1h before meals and hs) for 4-8wk. ***Maintenance:*** *Adult:* 1g BID.	B
Sulfacetamide ophthalmic *(Bleph-10, AK-Sulf, Sodium Sulamyd)*	*Sltn:* 10% in 5 and 15ml *Ointment:* 10% in 3.5g	*Adult:* **Sltn:** 1-2 drops Q 1-4h. **Ointment:** Apply 0.5 inch TID-QD.	C

Medication	Preparation	Dosing	Pregnancy Risk
Sulfadiazine (*Microsulfon*)	*Tab:* 500mg	Dosage varies with disease. ***Toxoplasmosis:*** see pp. 138-139.	C
Sulfadoxine/ pyrimethamine (*Fansidar*)	*Tab:* Sulfadoxine 500mg, pyrimethamine 25mg	***Malaria attack: PO:*** single dose may be given in combination with quinine. *Child <4y.o.:* $^1/_2$ tab. *Child 4-8y.o.:* 1 tab. *Child 9-14y.o.:* 2 tabs. *Child >15y.o.-adult:* 2-3 tabs. ***Malaria prophylaxis: PO:*** may double dose below and give Q 2wk. *Child <4y.o.:* $^1/_4$ tab Q wk. *Child 4-8y.o.:* $^1/_2$ tab Q wk. *Child 9-14y.o.:* $^3/_4$ tab Q wk. *Child >15y.o.-adult:* 1 tab Q wk. *Take first dose 1-2d before departure to endemic area. Continue during stay and for 4-6wk after return.*	C
Sulfamethoxazole (*Gantanol*)	*Tab:* 500mg	***UTI:*** *Child >2mo.:* load with 50-60mg/kg load, then 25-30mg/kg Q 12h.	C,D9
Sulfasalazine (*Azulfidine*)	*Tab:* 500mg *Tab EC:* 500mg	***Ulcerative colitis, mild to moderate:*** *Child >2y.o.:* start 40-60mg/kg/d in 4-6 divided doses, taper with response to 7.5mg/kg (max 500mg) QID. *Adult:* start 3-4g/d in evenly divided doses TID-QID, taper with response to 500mgQID.	B,D9
Sulfisoxazole (*Gantrisin*)	*Liquid:* 500mg/5ml *Tab:* 500mg	*Child >2mo.:* first dose 75mg/kg, then 37.5mg/kg (max 1.5g) Q 6h. *Adult:* initial dose 2-4g, then 1-2g Q 6h.	C,D9

See index for proprietary names of generic meds

Drug	Forms	Dosage	
Sulindac *(Clinoril)*	*Tab:* 150, 200mg	*Adult:* 150-200mg Q 12h.	B,D2-3
Sumatriptan *(Imitrex)*	*Nasal spray:* 5, 20mg *Tab:* 25, 50, 100mg *Inj:* 12mg/vial; 6mg/ml syringe	**Migraine HA: Nasal spray:** *Child >16y.o.-adult:* 5-20mg in one nostril. If no response after 2h, may repeat, max dose 40 mg/d. **PO:** *Child >16y.o.-adult:* initial dose 25mg (max 100mg). No evidence that initial dose of 100mg provides more relief than 25mg. If no response after 2h, may give 2nd dose up to 100mg. Repeat at 2h intervals, max 200mg/d. **SC:** *Child >16y.o.- adult:* 6mg. No evidence 2nd injection works if 1st fails. Max 2 doses (12mg)/24h must be at least 1h apart. *Do not use within 24h of ergotamine.*	C
Tacrine *(Cognex)*	*Cap:* 10, 20, 30, 40mg	**Alzheimer's:** *Adult:* start 10mg QID. After 4wk, dose may be increased to 20mg QID. Titrate to higher doses, up to 30-40mg QID, waiting 4wk before each increase as tolerated.	C
Tadalafil *(Cialis)*	*Tab:* 5, 10, 30mg	Adult male: 5-30mg (usually 10mg) 30min before sexual activity, max QD.	B
Tamoxifen *(Nolvadex)*	*Tab:* 10, 20mg	Adult: 20-40mg/d. Give QD if dose ≤20mg/d; give in divided doses BID if dose >20mg/d.	D
Tegaserod *(Zelnorm)*	*Tab:* 2, 6mg	Adult female *<65y.o: Irritable bowel syndrome:* 6mg BID before meals for 4-6wk.	B

Medication	Preparation	Dosing	Pregnancy Risk
Telithromycin (Ketek)	Tab: 400mg	Adult: 800mg po QD for 5-7d.	C
Telmisartan (Micardis)	Tab: 20, 40, 80mg	HTN: Adult: 40-80mg QD. If on a diuretic, start at 20mg QD.	C,D2-3
Tenecteplase (TNKase)	Vial: 50mg	Acute MI: Adult: give IV over 5sec. Dosing: <60kg: 30mg; 60-70kg: 35mg; 70-80kg: 40mg; 80-90kg: 45mg; >90kg: 50mg.	C
Tenofovir (Viread)	Tab: 300mg	Adult: 300mg Q 24h. "CrCl" <50, >30: 300mg Q 48h; "CrCl" <30, >10: 300mg twice a week.	B
Terazosin (Hytrin)	Tab: 1, 2, 5, 10mg Cap: 1, 2, 5, 10mg	HTN: Adult: initial dose 1mg hs. Usual dosing range 1-5mg/d, but doses up to 20mg/d used - give large doses QD or divide BID. BPH: Adult: initial dose 1mg hs. Titrate dose stepwise from 1-2mg up to 5-10mg/d to achieve desired results.	C
Terbinafine (Lamisil)	Cream 1%: 15-30g Tab: 250mg Spray: 1%	Child >12y.o.-adult: Tinea pedis, tinea cruris, tinea corporis: apply cream or spray to affected and surrounding area BID for 7-25d. Onychomycosis: Fingernail: 250mg po QD for 6wk. Toenail: 250mg po QD for 12wk.	B
Terbutaline (Brethine, Bricanyl)	Tab: 2.5, 5mg Inhaler: 200µg/puff Inj: 1mg/ml (1:1000)	PO: Child <12y.o.: start 0.05mg/kg TID, increase as needed to 0.15mg/kg TID, max 5mg/d. Child 12-15y.o.: 2.5mg TID. Child >15y.o.-adult: 5mg TID.	B

	Inhaler: *Child >12y.o.-adult:* 2 puffs Q 4-6h. **Nebulization:** *Child <2y.o.:* 0.5mg in 2.5ml NS. *Child 2-9y.o.:* 1mg in 2.5ml NS. *Child >9y.o.-adult:* 1.5mg in 2.5ml NS. **SC:** *Child <12y.o.:* 0.005-0.01mg/kg (max 0.25mg), may repeat in 15-20min. *Child >12y.o.-adult:* 0.25mg, may repeat in 15-30min.	
Terconazole *(Terazol 3, Terazol 7)*	*Vag cream:* 0.4% (Terazol 7) or 0.8% (Terazol 3) in tubes with applicator *Vag supp:* 80mg (Terazol 3)	*Adult:* 1 full applicator or suppository (0.8% cream or vag supp) intravaginally hs for 3d, or 1 full applicator (0.4% cream) hs for 7d.	C
Tetanus immune globulin *(Hyper-Tet)*	*Inj:* 250U/vial	***Prevention:*** *Child/adult:* 250-500U IM. Also see p. 46. ***Treatment:*** *Child/adult:* 3000-6000U IM. *Give at different site from toxoid.*	C
Tetracaine ophthalmic *(Pontocaine HCl)*	*Sltn:* 0.5% in 2 and 15ml	*Adult:* 1-2 drops. Not for prolonged use.	NR
Tetracycline	*Liquid:* 125mg/5ml *Tab:* 250, 500mg *Cap:* 100, 250, 500mg	*Child >8y.o.:* 6-12mg/kg (max 500mg) Q 6h. *Adult:* 250-500mg Q 6h.	D

Medication	Preparation	Dosing	Pregnancy Risk
Tetrahydrozoline nasal *(Tyzine)*	*Sltn:* 0.05%, 0.1%	*Child 2-6y.o.:* 2-3 drops 0.05% sltn each nostril. *Child 6y.o-adult:* 2-4 drops 0.1% sltn each nostril. Use Q 4-6h for 3-5d only.	C
Tetrahydrozoline ophthalmic *(Visine, Murine Plus)*	*Sltn:* 0.05% in 15 and 30ml	*Child/adult:* 1-2 drops each eye up to QID for 3-4d only.	C
Thiabendazole *(Mintezol)*	*Liquid:* 500mg/5ml *Tab (chew):* 500mg	*Child/adult:* 25mg/kg (max 1500mg) BID with food. **Strongyloides, ascariasis, uncinariasis, trichuriasis:** 2d. **Cutaneous larva migrans:** 2d. If active lesions still present 2d after treatment is complete, give 2nd course. **Trichinosis:** 2-4d. **Visceral larva migrans:** 7d.	C
Thiamine (Vitamin B1)	*Tab:* 50, 100, 250, 500mg *Thimilate EC: Tab:* 20mg *Inj:* 100mg/ml	**Wernicke's encephalopathy:** *Adult:* 100mg IV, then 100mg IV/IM QD for 3d. **Wet beriberi (with cardiac failure):** *Adult:* 10-30mg IV TID. **Beriberi:** *Adult:* 10-20mg IM TID for 2wk, then MVI (containing 5-10mg thiamine) QD for 1mo.	A,C[§]

Drug	Forms	Dosing	
Thiethylperazine *(Torecan, Norzine)*	*Tab:* 10mg *Supp:* 10mg *Inj:* 5mg/ml	***Nausea/vomiting: PO/PR/IM:*** *Child >12y.o.- adult:* 10mg Q 8h prn.	NR
Thiopental *(Pentothal)*	*Syringes:* 0.25, 0.4, 0.5, 1.0, 2.5g	***Rapid-sequence intubation:*** *Child/adult:* 2-5mg/kg IV. *Use smaller dose if patient at risk for hemodynamic compromise. See p. 15 for rapid-sequence intubation protocol.*	C
Thioridazine *(Mellaril)*	*Concentrate:* 30, 100mg/ml *Liquid:* 25, 100mg/ml *Tab:* 10, 25, 50, 100, 150, 200mg	*Child 2-12y.o.:* 0.5-3mg/kg/d divided BID-QID. *Adult:* start 25-100mg TID, usual range 150-800mg/d divided BID-QID.	C
Thiothixene *(Navane)*	*Concentrate:* 5mg/ml *Cap:* 1, 2, 5, 10, 20mg *Inj:* 2, 5mg/ml	**PO:** *Adult:* 6-60mg/d, divided BID-TID. **IM:** *Adult:* 4mg BID-QID. Usual range 16-20 mg/d, max 30mg/d.	C
Tiagabine *(Gabitril)*	*Tab:* 2, 4, 12, 16mg	**Seizures:** *Child 12-18y.o.:* 4-32mg/d. *Adult:* 4-56mg/d. Give 4mg/d QD, larger doses BID-QID, depending on dose.	C

Medication	Preparation	Dosing	Pregnancy Risk
Ticarcillin *(Ticar)*	*Inj:* 1, 3, 6g	*Neonates: <2kg, <7d:* 75mg/kg IM/IV Q 12h. *<2kg, >7d:* 75mg/kg IM/IV Q 8h. *>2kg, <7d:* 75mg/kg IM/IV Q 8h. *>2kg, >7d:* 100mg/kg IM/IV Q 8h. *Child <40kg:* 200-300mg/kg/d IM/IV divided Q 4-6h, max 18g/d. *Child >40kg-adult:* 3g Q 4h or 4g Q 6h IM/IV, max 18g/d. *Max IM dose 2g.*	B
Ticarcillin/ clavulanate *(Timentin)*	*Inj:* Ticarcillin 3g/clavulanic acid 0.1g	*IV: Child <1wk, <2kg:* 75mg/kg Q 12h. *Child <1wk, >2kg:* 75mg/kg Q 8h. *Child 1wk-3mo., <2kg:* 75mg/kg Q 8h. *Child 1wk-3mo., >2kg:* 75mg/kg Q 6h. *Child >3mo., <60kg:* 200-300mg/kg/d divided Q 4-6h, max 24g/d. *Child ≥60kg-adult:* 3.1g Q 4-6h.	B
Ticlopidine *(Ticlid)*	*Tab:* 250mg	*Adult:* 250mg BID with food. *Associated with neutropenia.*	B
Timolol *(Blocadren)*	*Tab:* 5, 10, 20mg	*HTN: Adult:* initial dose 10mg BID. Usual maintenance 10-20mg (max 30mg) BID. *Post MI: Adult:* 10mg BID. *Migraine: Adult:* 10mg BID.	C,D2-3
Timolol ophthalmic *(Betimol, Timoptic)*	*Sltn:* 0.25% and 0.5% in 2.5, 5, 10, and 15ml	*Glaucoma: Adult:* 1 drop in affected eye QD-BID.	C

See index for proprietary names of generic meds

Drug	Form	Dose	Category
Tinzaparin *(Innohep)*	*Inj:* 20,000IU/ml	***DVT/PE:*** *Adult:* 175IU/kg SC QD for at least 6d. ***Prophylaxis DVT:*** *Adult:* 50IU/kg SC QD.	B
Tioconazole *(Monistat 1, Vagistat-1)*	*Vag ointment:* 6.5% in 4.6g applicator	*Adult:* 1 full applicator hs once only.	C
Tiotropium *(Spiriva)*	*Inh:* 18µg	*Adult:* 18µg inhaled QD.	C
Tirofiban *(Aggrastat)*	*Inj:* 50, 250µg/ml	*Adult:* 0.4µg/kg/min for 30min, then 0.1µg/kg/min infusion for 12-24h post-procedure. Patients with CrCl <30 ml/min: halve dose.	B
Tobramycin *(Nebcin)*	*Inj:* 40mg/ml	**IM/IV:** *Child <1wk:* 1.3-2mg/kg Q 12h. *Child >1wk-1mo.:* 2-2.5mg/kg Q 8h. *Child >1mo.:* 1.5-2mg/kg Q 8h. **Cystic fibrosis:** 2.5mg/kg IV Q 6h. *Adult:* load 2mg/kg, then 1.7mg/kg Q 8h. Alternate QD dosing (only if adult <75y.o. with creat <1.5): 4-7mg/kg. Adjust for renal function, check levels.	D
Tobramycin ophthalmic *(Tobrex)*	*Sltn:* 0.3% *Ointment:* 3mg/g	*Adult:* Sltn: 1-2 drops Q 2-4h. Ointment: apply BID-TID.	C
Tocainide *(Tonocard)*	*Tab:* 400, 600mg	*Adult:* ***Ventricular arrhythmias:*** 400-800mg Q 8h. ***Myotonic dystrophy:*** 800-1200mg/d.	C

Medication	Preparation	Dosing	Pregnancy Risk
Tolazamide *(Tolinase)*	*Tab:* 100, 250, 500mg	*Adult (FBS ≤200mg/dl or ≥65y.o.):* start 100mg QD with breakfast. *Adult (FBS >200mg/dl or <65y.o.):* start 250mg QD, max 500mg BID with meals.	C
Tolbutamide *(Orinase)*	*Tab:* 500mg	*Adult:* start 1-2g QD or divided BID, max 3g/d.	C
Tolmetin *(Tolectin)*	*Tab:* 200, 600mg *Cap:* 400mg	*Child >2y.o.:* start 7mg/kg TID, then give 5-10mg/kg TID. *Adult:* start 400mg TID, titrate to max 600-1800mg/d divided TID.	C,D3
Tolterodine *(Detrol)*	*Tab:* 1, 2mg *Tab LA:* 2, 4mg	*Adult:* **Tab:** 1-2mg BID. **Tab LA:** 2-4mg QD.	C
Topiramate *(Topamax)*	*Tab:* 25, 100, 200mg *Cap:* 15, 25mg	*Adult:* start 50mg/d, titrate. Usual dose is 200mg po BID. *Adjust dosage for renal insufficiency.*	C
Torsemide *(Demadex)*	*Tab:* 5, 10, 20, 100mg *Inj:* 10mg/ml	*Adult:* **HTN:** 5-10mg po QD. **CHF:** start 10-20mg po/IV. **CRF:** starting dose 20mg po/IV. **Cirrhosis:** start 5-10mg po/IV, max dose 40mg. *Double ineffective doses. Begin with lower doses. Max po/IV dose = 200mg. Oral dosing is equipotent with IV doses.*	B
Tramadol *(Ultram)*	*Tab:* 50mg	*Adult:* 25-100mg Q 4-6h prn for pain, max 400mg/d. *Adult >75y.o.:* max 300mg/d divided Q 4-6h.	C

See index for proprietary names of generic meds

Trandolapril *(Mavik)*	*Tab:* 1, 2, 4mg	*Adult:* initial 1-2mg QD. Increase dose Q wk to 2-4mg/d. 4mg/d may be given as 2mg BID. Max dose 8mg/d.	C,D2-3
Tranylcypromine *(Parnate)*	*Tab:* 10mg	*Adult:* 30-60mg/d divided BID-TID.	C
Travoprost *(Travatan)*	*Sltn:* 0.004%	*Adult:* 1 drop in affected eye qpm.	C
Trazodone *(Desyrel)*	*Tab:* 50, 100, 150mg	*Adult:* initial dose 75mg BID, increase by 50mg/d Q 3-4d, max outpatient dose 400mg/d, max inpatient dose 600mg/d. Divide BID-TID.	C
Treprostinil *(Remodulin)*	*Inj:* 1mg/ml, 2.5mg/ml, 5mg/ml, 10mg/ml	*Adult* pulmonary arterial HTN: 0.625-2.5ng/kg/ min; **AVOID** abrupt cessation.	B
Triamcinolone acetonide *(Aristocort, Azmacort, Kenalog, Nasacort)*	*Cream:* 0.025%, 0.1%, 0.5% *Inhalation:* 100µg/puff *Inj:* 40mg/ml *Spr:* 55µg/spray	**Dermatoses:** *Child:* 0.025% QD-BID or 0.1%-0.5% QD. *Adult:* BID-QID. **Asthma:** *Child 6-12y.o.:* 1-2 puffs 3 to 4 times/d or 2-4 puffs twice/d, max 12 sprays/24h. *Adult:* 2 puffs TID-QD or 4 puffs BID, max 16 puffs/24h. **Arthritic condition:** *>6y.o. and adult:* 2.5-15mg, may repeat as necessary. Adult adjust to 10-80mg/d as necessary. **Rhinitis, allergic:** *Child (>6y.o.) and adult:* initial: 2 sprays in each nostril QD; maintenance: 1 spray in each nostril QD.	C

Medication	Preparation	Dosing	Pregnancy Risk
Triamterene *(Dyrenium)*	*Cap:* 50, 100mg	*Adult:* initial 100mg BID after meals, max 300mg/d.	C,D(Htn)
Triazolam *(Halcion)*	*Tab:* 0.125, 0.25, 0.5mg	*Adult <65y.o.:* 0.125-0.5mg hs for up to 2-3wk. *Adult >65y.o.:* 0.125-0.25mg hs for up to 2-3wk. To DC, reduce dose by 50% Q 2 nights till 0.125mg for 2 nights, then DC.	X
Trifluoperazine *(Stelazine)*	*Liquid:* 10mg/ml *Tab:* 1, 2, 5, 10, 20mg *Inj:* 2mg/ml	*Child 6-12y.o.:* **PO/IM:** start 1mg QD-BID, usual max 15mg/d. *Adult:* **PO:** start 2-5mg po QD-BID, usual range 15-20mg/d, max 40mg/d. **IM:** 1-2mg Q 4-6h prn.	C
Trifluridine ophthalmic *(Viroptic)*	*Sltn:* 1% in 7.5ml	***Keratitis:*** *Adult:* 1 drop Q 2h while awake (5-9 drops/d). Following re-epithelialization, 1 drop Q 4h for 7d, max 21d total.	NR
Trihexyphenidyl *(Artane)*	*Liquid:* 2mg/5ml *Tab:* 2, 5mg *Cap SR:* 5mg	*Adult:* start 1-2mg/d, titrate to up to 15mg/d, divide TID. SR caps are for pts on stable dosing; convert on mg per mg basis and give QD after breakfast or BID with meals.	C
Trimethobenzamide *(Tigan)*	*Cap:* 100, 250mg *Supp (pediatric):* 100mg *Supp:* 200mg *Inj:* 100mg/ml	**PO:** *Child 15-40kg:* 100-200mg TID-QID. *Child >40kg-adult:* 250mg TID-QID. **Rectal:** *Child <15kg:* 100mg TID-QID. *Child >15kg:* 100-200mg TID-QID. *Adult:* 200mg TID-QID. **IM:** *Adult:* 200mg TID-QID.	C

See index for proprietary names of generic meds

Trimethoprim (*Trimpex, Proloprim*)	*Tab:* 100, 200mg	*Adult:* 100mg Q 12h or 200mg QD for 10d.	C
Trimethoprim/ sulfamethoxazole (*Bactrim, Septra*)	*Liquid:* Trimeth 40mg/Sulf 200mg per 5ml *Tab:* Trimeth 80mg/Sulf 400mg (SS); Trimeth 160mg/Sulf 800mg (DS) *Inj:* Trimeth 16mg/Sulf 80mg per ml	***Pneumocystis pneumonia:*** see p. xxx. ***Minor infection:*** *Child >2mo.:* as trimeth 4-5mg/kg po/IV Q 12h. *(Easy po dosing = 0.5ml liquid/kg po BID.) Adult:* as trimeth 160mg (=1DS tab) po/IV Q 12h. ***Severe infection:*** *Child >2mo.-adult:* as trimeth 15-20mg/kg/d po/IV divided Q 6-8h. ***Acute bronchitis:*** 1 DS tab Q 12h for 14d. ***Traveler's diarrhea:*** *Adult:* 1 DS tab Q 12h for 5d.	C
Trimetrexate (*NeuTrexin*)	*Inj:* 25, 200mg vials	***Pneumocystis pneumonia:*** see pp. 129-130. *Adult:* 45mg/m^2 QD IV infusion over 60-90min for 21d. *Leucovorin must be given along with trimetrexate for 24d.*	D
Trimipramine (*Surmontil*)	*Cap:* 25, 50, 100mg	*Adult outpatient:* 25-50mg TID, max 200mg/d. *Adult inpatient:* 50mg BID up to 100mg TID. *Start adolescents and elderly with 50mg/d.*	C

Medication	Preparation	Dosing	Pregnancy Risk
Tropicamide ophthalmic *(Mydriacyl, Tropicacyl)*	*Sltn:* 0.5% and 1% in 2, 5 and 15ml	***Examination of fundus:*** *Adult:* 15-20min before exam, instill 1-2 drops of 0.5% while compressing lacrimal sac.	C
Trospium *(Sanctura)*	*Tab:* 20mg	*Adult:* 20mg QD-BID at least 1h before meals.	NR
Urokinase *(Abbokinase)*	*Inj:* 250,000IU	***Pulmonary embolus:*** see pp. 132-133.	B
Valacyclovir *(Valtrex)*	*Tab:* 500mg, 1g	***Herpes zoster:*** 1g Q 8h for 7d. ***Initial episode genital herpes:*** 1g BID for 10d. ***Recurrent episode genital herpes:*** 500mg BID for 3d. ***Suppression of recurrent genital herpes:*** 1g QD. *Use valacyclovir for immunocompetent adults only.*	B
Valproate *(Depacon)*	*Inj:* 100mg/ml	***Seizures:*** *Child/adult:* 15-30mg/kg/d as an infusion over at least 60min, max rate 20mg/min.	D

See index for proprietary names of generic meds

Valproic acid (*Depakene*, *Depakote*)	Depakene: *Liquid:* 250mg/5ml *Cap:* 250mg Depakote: *Sprinkle cap:* 125mg *Tab:* 125, 250, 500mg Depakote ER: *Tab:* 250, 500mg	*Seizures: Child/adult* (Depakene, Depakote): 15-60mg/kg/d. Divide if dose exceeds 250mg/d. *Mania: Adult* (Depakote): start 375mg BID, max 60mg/kg/d. *Migraine HA: Adult:* (Depakote, Depakote ER): 250-500mg BID.	D
Valsartan (*Diovan*)	*Tab:* 40, 80, 160, 320mg	*HTN: Adult:* 80-320mg QD. *CHF:* start 40mg BID, usual maintenance 80-160mg BID.	C,D2-3
Vancomycin (*Vancocin*)	*Pulvules:* 125, 250mg *Oral sltn:* 1, 10g *Inj:* 0.5, 1, 5, 10g	*Meningitis:* see pp. 121-123. *IV: Child <1mo.:* initial dose 15mg/kg, then 10mg/kg Q 12h (*if <1wk old*) or Q 8h (*if ≥1wk old*). *Child >1mo.:* 10mg/kg Q 6h. *Adult:* 1g Q 12h.	B
Vardenifil (*Levitra*)	*Tab:* 2.5, 5, 10, 20mg	*Adult male:* 5-20mg (usually 10mg) 60min before sexual activity, max QD.	B
Vecuronium (*Norcuron*)	*Inj:* 10mg	*Child >7wk-adult:* 0.1mg/kg/dose.	C
Venlafaxine (*Effexor*)	*Tab:* 25, 37.5, 50, 75, 100mg *Cap XR:* 37.5, 75, 150mg	*Depression: Adult:* 75-225mg/d divided BID-TID with food. *Give XR form QD.*	C

Medication	Preparation	Dosing	Pregnancy Risk
Verapamil *(Calan, Isoptin, Verelan)*	*Tab: 40, 80, 120mg* *SR tab: 120, 180, 240mg* *SR cap: 120, 180, 240, 360mg* *Inj: 2.5mg/ml*	**PO: *HTN:*** *Child:* 4-10mg/kg/d. *Adult:* 240-480mg/d. Give tab TID, SR tab and SR cap QD. **Angina/prevention of PSVT:** 240-480mg/d, divided Q 6-8h. *Use tab only.* **Control of ventricular rate in atrial flutter/atrial fib:** 240-480mg/d, divided Q 6-8h. *Use tab only.* **IV:** *Give IV over 2min. May repeat once in 15-30min. Child <1y.o.:* 0.1-0.2mg/kg. *Child 1-15y.o.:* 0.1-0.3mg/kg (max 5mg 1st dose, 1mg 2nd dose). *Child 15y.o.-adult:* 5-10mg.	C
Vidarabine ophthalmic *(Vira-A)*	*Ointment: 3% in 3.5g*	***Keratitis:*** *Adult:* Apply 0.5inch 5 times/d at 3h intervals.	C
Vitamin K1 *(Phytonadione) (AquaMEPHYTON Mephyton)*	*Tab: 5mg* *Inj: 2, 10mg/ml*	***Oral anticoagulant overdose:*** *Infants:* **SC:** 1-2mg/dose Q 4-8h prn. *Child/Adult:* **PO/IV/SC:** 2.5-10mg/dose. May repeat in 6-8h if given IM, IV, SC; in 12-48h if po. *See page 80 for recommendations on therapeutic warfarin OD.*	C
Voriconizole *(VFEND)*	*Tab: 50, 200mg* *Inj: 200mg powder*	***Aspergillosis, invasive:*** *12y.o-adult:* 6mg/kg IV Q 12h, then 4mg/kg IV Q 12h. **Oral maintenance:** *<40kg:* 150-200mg Q 12h; *>40kg:* 200-300mg Q 12h.	D

Warfarin *(Coumadin)*	*Tab:* 1, 2, 2.5, 3, 4, 5, 6, 7.5, 10mg	*Dose varies with disease process and individual.* X
Zafirlukast *(Accolate)*	*Tab:* 10, 20mg	*Child 5-12y.o.:* 10mg BID. *Child >12y.o.-adult:* 20mg BID. Take 1h before or 2h after meals. B
Zalcitabine *(ddC)* *(Hivid)*	*Tab:* 0.375, 0.75mg	*Adult:* 0.75mg Q 8h. *If CrCl 10-40ml/min:* 0.75mg Q 12h. *If CrCl <10ml/min:* 0.75mg Q 24h. C
Zaleplon *(Sonata)*	*Tab:* 5, 10mg	*Adult:* usual dose 10mg hs, consider 5mg in elderly or low-weight individuals. *Max dose:* 20mg. C
Zidovudine *(Retrovir)*	*Liquid:* 50mg/5ml *Tab:* 300mg *Cap:* 100mg *Inj:* 10mg/ml	**PO:** *Child 3mo.-12y.o.:* 180mg/m² (max 200mg) Q 8h. *Child >12y.o.-adult:* 300mg BID. **IV:** *Adult:* 1-2mg/kg over 1h Q 4h. **Prevention of maternal-fetal HIV transmission:** *Maternal dosing:* after 14th wk of preg, 100mg po 5 times/d until labor, then during L&D: load 2mg/kg IV over 1h, followed by 1mg/kg/h infusion until clamping of umbilical cord. *Neonatal dosing:* 2mg/kg po Q 6h (within 12h after birth up to 6wk of age). *If unable to take po, 1.5mg/kg IV Q 6h.* C
Zileuton *(Zyflo)*	*Tab:* 600mg	**Asthma:** *Child >12y.o.-adult:* 600mg QID with meals and hs. C
Ziprasidone *(Geodon)*	*Tab:* 20, 40, 60, 80mg *Inj:* 20mg	**PO:** *Adult:* start 20mg BID, maintenance 20-100mg BID. **IM:** *Adult:* 10mg Q 2h or 20mg IM Q 4h, max 40mg/d. C

Medication	Preparation	Dosing	Pregnancy Risk
Zoledronic acid (*Zometa*)	*Inj:* 4mg powder	*Adult:* 4mg IV ×1, may repeat in 7d.	D
Zolmitriptan (*Zomig*)	*Nasal spray:* 5mg/spray *Tab:* 2.5, 5mg	*Adult:* 1.25-5mg po or 1 nasal spray at onset of sx, may repeat in 2h, max 10mg/d.	C
Zolpidem (*Ambien*)	*Tab:* 5, 10mg	*Adult:* 5-10mg hs. *Start at lower doses for elderly or debilitated patients.*	B
Zonisamide (*Zonegran*)	*Cap:* 100mg	*Adult:* 100-600mg/d QD or divided BID.	C

See index for proprietary names of generic meds

Major references are in **bold type**; proprietary names are in *italic type*. Page numbers followed by "f" indicate figures.

Pediatric Visual Acuity Chart

(Adult chart on reverse)
Test distance 13 inches

20/200

20/160

20/100

20/80

    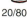

20/60

20/40

        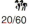

20/30

  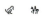

323

Adult Visual Acuity Chart

(Pediatric chart on reverse)

Test distance 14 inches

8 4	✈	20/800
5 9	✈ ✈	20/400
7 3 6 2	✈ ✈ ✈	20/200
8 2 4 6 7	✈ ✈ ✈	20/100
6 7 5 3 9 4	✈ ✈ ✈	20/70
2 6 4 8 5 3	✈ ✈ ✈	20/50
5 7 8 3 6 9	✈ ✈ ✈	20/40
8 3 2 5 9 4	✈ ✈ ✈	20/30
3 4 5 7 6 8	✈ ✈ ✈	20/25
9 3 7 4 2 6	✈ ✈ ✈	20/20